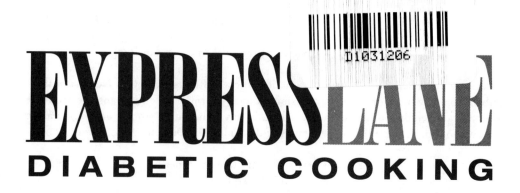

DIABETIC COOKING

ROBYN WEBB

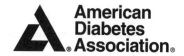

American Diabetes Association

Director, Book Publishing, John Fedor; *Editor,* Aime Ballard-Wood; *Production Manager,* Peggy M. Rote; *Composition,* Circle Graphics; *Cover Design,* VC Graphics Design Studio; *Nutrient Analysis,* Nutritional Computing Consultants, Inc.; *Printer,* Sheridan Books.

Printed in the United States of America
1 3 5 7 9 10 8 6 4 2

The suggestions and information contained in this publication are generally consistent with the *Clinical Practice Recommendations* and other policies of the American Diabetes Association, but they do not represent the policy or position of the Association or any of its boards or committees. Reasonable steps have been taken to ensure the accuracy of the information presented. However, the American Diabetes Association cannot ensure the safety or efficacy of any product or service described in this publication. Individuals are advised to consult a physician or other appropriate health care professional before undertaking any diet or exercise program or taking any medication referred to in this publication. Professionals must use and apply their own professional judgment, experience, and training and should not rely solely on the information contained in this publication before prescribing any diet, exercise, or medication. The American Diabetes Association—its officers, directors, employees, volunteers, and members—assumes no responsibility or liability for personal or other injury, loss, or damage that may result from the suggestions or information in this publication.

♾ The paper in this publication meets the requirements of the ANSI Standard Z39.48-1992 (permanence of paper).

ADA titles may be purchased for business or promotional use or for special sales. For information, please write to Lee Romano Sequeira, Special Sales & Promotions, at the address below.

American Diabetes Association
1701 North Beauregard Street
Alexandria, VA 22311

Library of Congress Cataloging-in-Publication Data

Webb, Robyn.
    Express lane diabetic cooking / Robyn Webb.
        p. cm.
    ISBN 1-58040-005-1 (pbk. : alk. paper)
    1. Diabetes—Diet therapy—Recipes.   2. Quick and easy cookery.   3. Convenience foods.   I. Title.

    RC662.W3556 2000
    641.5'6314—dc21

                                                            00-56551

To my husband, Allan, and my mother, Ruth. Thanks for your support.

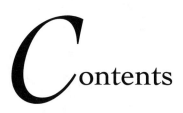

Contents

A Note about Food Labels

MANY FOOD LABELS IN THE GROCERY STORE use terms that can be confusing. To help you shop and eat better, here is a list of the common terms as defined by the Food and Drug Administration.

Sugar

Sugar Free: Less than 0.5 gram of sugar per serving.
No Added Sugar, Without Added Sugar, No Sugar Added: This does not mean the same as "sugar free." A label bearing these words means that no sugars were added during processing, or that processing does not increase the sugar content above the amount the ingredients naturally contain. Consult the nutrition information panel to see the total amount of sugar in this product.
Reduced Sugar: At least 25% less sugar per serving than the regular product.

Calories

Calorie Free: Fewer than 5 calories per serving.
Low Calorie: 40 calories or less per serving. (If servings are smaller than 30 grams, or smaller than 2 tablespoons, this means 40 calories or less per 50 grams of food.)
Reduced Calorie, Fewer Calories: At least 25% fewer calories per serving than the regular product.

Fat

Fat Free, Nonfat: Less than 0.5 gram of fat per serving.
Low Fat: 3 grams or less of fat per serving. (If servings are smaller than 30 grams, or smaller than 2 tablespoons, this means 3 grams or less of fat per 50 grams of food.)
Reduced Fat, Less Fat: At least 25% less fat per serving than the regular product.

Cholesterol

Cholesterol Free: Less than 2 milligrams of cholesterol, and 2 grams or less of saturated fat per serving.
Low Cholesterol: 20 milligrams or less of cholesterol, and 2 grams or less of saturated fat per serving.
Reduced Cholesterol, Less Cholesterol: At least 25% less cholesterol, and 2 grams or less of saturated fat per serving than the regular product.

Sodium

Sodium Free: Less than 5 milligrams of sodium per serving.
Low Sodium: 140 milligrams or less of sodium per serving.
Very Low Sodium: 35 milligrams or less of sodium per serving.
Reduced Sodium, Less Sodium: At least 25% less sodium per serving than the regular product.

Light or Lite Foods

Foods that are labeled "Light" or "Lite" are usually either lower in fat or lower in calories than the regular product. Some products may also be lower in sodium. Check the nutrition information label on the back of the product to make sure.

Meat and Poultry

Lean: Less than 10 grams of fat, 4.5 grams or less of saturated fat, and less than 95 milligrams of cholesterol per serving and per 100 grams.
Extra Lean: Less than 5 grams of fat, less than 2 grams of saturated fat, and less than 95 milligrams of cholesterol per serving and per 100 grams.

A Note from the American Diabetes Association

THERE IS A PRICE TO PAY for using convenience foods in a recipe: high sodium content, sometimes way beyond the total daily recommended amount! If you are watching your sodium intake, check each recipe for its sodium content to make sure you can safely work it into your meal plan. Remember, you can always reduce the sodium content of a recipe with deli meats by using the plain, cooked version of the meat (plain roasted chicken or turkey instead of smoked from the deli). You may be able to find broth with no added sodium instead of the low-sodium variety used here, and lower-sodium canned tomato products. If a recipe calls for added salt, you could use a salt substitute. You know the drill!

Regarding the nutrient analysis, unless otherwise indicated, the first of alternative choices listed in a recipe was used. If a food or seasoning is called for "to taste," it is not included in the analysis. If a food is listed as "optional," it is not included in the analysis. Finally, if a serving suggestion appears in the last line of the directions instead of the ingredient list, that food is not included in the analysis.

Bon appetit!

Acknowledgments

PERHAPS IN NO OTHER ASPECT OF MY CAREER have I experienced the concept of teamwork more than when I write books. I'd like to thank my team at the American Diabetes Association: Rob Anthony, my culinary buddy; Aime Ballard-Wood and Laurie Guffey, my expert editors; Peggy Rote, who always answers my questions; and Peter Banks, who provides consistent support and encouragement. Special gratitude to Jill Crum and Austin Zakari for their great work on the deli and frozen food sections of this book. Their love of good food really shines through. Finally, I appreciate my clients, people with diabetes and those without, who continue to inspire me to create recipes that are healthy, but most importantly, taste delicious!

Robyn Webb

*I*ntroduction

PICTURE THIS. IT'S LATE, YOU COME HOME FROM WORK, and there's nothing in your kitchen to put together a decent meal. Or so you think! With a little help from the salad bar, deli department, frozen food aisle, and other quick items from your supermarket, dinner can be minutes away. Many of the recipes here will take less than 20 minutes to prepare. Some of the recipes have no more than 5 ingredients. But since the ready-made ingredients are paired with fresh foods, each dish tastes like it was made from scratch. No one will know that Asian Coleslaw was made from prepackaged shredded cabbages and a few bottled condiments or that Spicy Summer Gazpacho was created from salad bar vegetables and shelf-stable spicy tomato juice.

Once you are hooked on the idea of saving time using prepackaged foods, you modify some of your other time-consuming recipes. With a properly-stocked pantry and a quick weekly trip to the store, you'll be able to whip up fast, easy meals that taste great, too. You'll use the ideas here for years to come.

This book presents chapters of recipes from four basic sections of the market: salad bar, deli, frozen foods, and aisles stocking shelf-stable items like beans, pasta, and rice. Then you add in supporting foods from the produce, dairy, and seafood departments. You can think of your supermarket as divided into these four major areas with support from the other three.

Each recipe tells you which sections of the store you need to visit to purchase the ingredients. When you can't find an ingredient in your store, the recipe gives you an alternative. For example, if diced zucchini is not at your salad bar, go to the produce department and prepare the zucchini according to the recipe. And you still have a choice about which section of the market your main ingredients come from. For instance, you can buy fresh chicken from the meat department, frozen chicken breasts, or smoked, cooked slices from the deli to use in any recipe calling for chicken. It may take a little longer to cook the chicken or defrost the breasts, but you may be able to better meet the goals of your individual meal plan. The choice is up to you.

A few notes about the recipes. I use mostly olive and canola oils. Keep your oils stored in a cool, dry, dark place. Prolonged exposure to heat and light will cause the oil to become rancid faster. You can fill a pump spray bottle with olive oil flavored with herbs and mist it over salad or popcorn. Use fresh ground pepper to bring out the best flavor in the recipes. Since many of the vegetables are prechopped, be sure to use them up quickly. Prolonged exposure to light and air will cause the vegetables to lose nutrition and flavor. Also, anything you buy from the frozen foods department should be free of ice crystals. Ice crystals indicate that the food was thawed and refrozen. Try and keep frozen foods no longer than three to six months (see the chart on freezing and storage of foods, page 10).

Stocking Your Pantry

Keeping common shelf-stable items in your pantry will save you hours of accumulated shopping time. Although it is important to have the items on this pantry list on hand, don't overstock. Items stocked in an overcrowded pantry are seldom found. Here's what you should have on hand to avoid a last-minute trip to the market.

Herbs and Spices

Be sure to use these up within a year. After that they are still safe to use, but their flavor fades considerably. Keep dried spices and herbs away from the heat. This includes storing them near the stove or near the refrigerator (yes, the fridge gives off heat!). Some people like to store their spices and herbs in a drawer in one single layer so they can find what they need quickly.

allspice
basil
bay leaves

chili powder
cinnamon
cloves

cumin
curry powder
dry mustard
garlic bulb
Italian seasoning
marjoram
nutmeg
onion powder
oregano

paprika
peppercorns
rosemary
saffron
sage
sea salt
sesame seeds
thyme
turmeric

Canned Products, Condiments, Vinegars, and Oils

Worcestershire sauce
lite soy sauce
low-sodium teriyaki sauce
sugar-free jams and jellies
low-fat Marinara sauce
white wine vinegar
red wine vinegar
balsamic vinegar
olive oil
canola oil
sesame oil
salsa
low-fat mayonnaise
Dijon mustard

low-fat, low-sodium chicken
    and beef broth
canned tomatoes
tomato paste
crushed tomatoes
white meat tuna
fat-free Italian salad dressing
fat-free refried beans
black olives
hoisin sauce
pesto
sun-dried tomatoes (not in oil)
capers

Grains, Pastas, and Beans

Keep flours, pastas, and grains in well-sealed containers. You
may also place these items in the refrigerator if you have room.

all-purpose flour
whole-wheat flour

pasta: spaghetti, bow-tie noodles,
    vermicelli, linguine, angel hair
couscous

white rice

brown rice

jasmine rice

tortillas

whole-wheat pita bread

beans: chickpeas (garbanzo),
pinto, black, red kidney, navy

Selecting and Storing Fruits and Vegetables

Although you may choose to use the produce called for in this book from the salad bar, not every supermarket will supply what you need. Therefore, below is handy info to help you select and store the most common fruits and vegetables.

Apples. Fruit should be firm and of good color for the variety. Any apple can be used for any purpose, but results vary. Keep cold and humid. Available all year.

Avocados. Color ranges from purple to black to green according to variety. Irregular brown marks on surface are superficial and don't affect the quality. Hold at room temperature until fruit yields gently to pressure, then refrigerate. Available all year.

Bananas. Fruit should be plump. Color varies from green to dark yellow with brownish flecks, according to degree of ripeness. Avoid grayish-yellow fruit; this indicates chilling injury. Ripen at room temperature. When at the stage of preferred ripeness, eat or refrigerate. Skin color turns brown, but flesh keeps well for several days. Available all year.

Berries. Choose plump, firm, full-colored berries. All varieties, with the exception of strawberries, should be free of their hull. Avoid any baskets showing signs of bruised or leaking fruit. Cover and refrigerate. Use within a few days. Available mainly June to August.

Cantaloupes. They should be fresh of any stem and give when pressed gently. Hold at room temperature for a few days, then refrigerate and use as soon as possible. Available mainly May to September.

Cherries. Sweet cherries are bright and glossy, ranging from deep red to black in color. They should be attached to fresh, green stems. Avoid cherries that are hard, sticky, or light in color. Refrigerate and use within a few days. Available May to August.

Coconuts. Choose nuts that are heavy for their size and full of liquid. Keep cold. Available all year, with a peak from September to January.

Cranberries. Select plump, firm, lustrous red to reddish-black berries. Refrigerate and use within two weeks. Can be frozen in original package. Available September to December.

Dates. Fruit should be soft and a lustrous brown. After package is opened, refrigerate. Keep then well wrapped to avoid drying and hardening. Available all year.

Grapefruit. Should be firm, not puffy or loose-skinned. Look for globular fruits that are heavy for their size, indicating juiciness. Green tinge does not affect eating quality. Refrigerate or keep at room temperature. Available all year.

Grapes. Choose plump, well-colored grapes that are firmly attached to green, pliable stems. Green grapes are sweetest when yellow-green in color. Red varieties are best when rich, red color predominates. Grapes won't increase in sweetness, so there's no need to hold them for further ripening. Refrigerate and use within one week. Available June through February.

Honeydew Melons. Look for a creamy or yellowish-white rind with a velvety feel. Avoid stark-white or greenish tinged rinds. Hold at room temperature for a few days, then refrigerate. Peak: June to October.

Lemons and Limes. Look for a fine-textured skin indicating juiciness. Select those that are heavy for their size. Keep at room temperature or refrigerate. Available all year.

Mangos. Skin color generally green with yellowish to red areas. Red and yellow color increases with ripening. Avoid any having grayish skin discoloration, pitting, or black spots. Keep at room temperature until soft. When fully soft, refrigerate. Peak May to August.

Oranges. Should be firm and heavy with a fine-textured skin. In some varieties, a green skin color does not affect eating quality. Store at room temperature or refrigerate. Available all year.

Papayas. Select medium-sized, well-colored fruit, that is, at least half yellow. Ripen at room temperature until skin color is primarily golden, then refrigerate. Peak October to December.

Peaches and Nectarines. Glowing blush is not a true indication of ripeness. Background color of peaches should be yellowish or cream colored; nectarines are yellow-orange when ripe. Fruit should be firm with a slight softening along the seam line. Avoid green or greenish-tinged fruits and any that are hard, dull, or bruised. Peak June to September.

Pears. Color varies according to variety. Pears generally require additional ripening at home. Hold at room temperature until stem end yields to gentle pressure, then refrigerate. Year-round availability of different varieties.

Persimmons. Look for plump, smooth, highly colored fruit with a green cap. Keep at room temperature until soft. When ripe, refrigerate. Peak October to December.

Pineapple. Select large fruit having fresh green leaves. Shell color is not an indicator of maturity. Store upside-down to ripen or eat immediately. Keep at room temperature or refrigerate. Available year-round. Peak March to June.

Plums. Appearance and flavor differ widely by variety. Hold at room temperature until they yield gently to pressure. Peak June to September.

Pomegranates. Rind should be pink or bright red with a crimson seeded flesh. Avoid any that appear dry. Keep cold and humid. Available September to November.

Strawberries. Choose berries that are fresh, clean, bright, and red. The green caps should be intact and the fruit should be free of bruises. Strawberries are best eaten immediately but if they must be stored, refrigerate them with their caps intact. Available year-round. Peak April through June.

Tangelos. Look for firm, thin-skinned fruits that are heavy for their size. Keep at room temperature or refrigerate. Available October to January.

Tangerines. Choose fruit heavy for its size. A puffy appearance and feel is normal. Refrigerate and use as soon as possible. Peak November to January.

Watermelons. Difficult to determine ripeness of uncut melons. Choose firm, smooth melons with a waxy bloom or dullness on the rind. Underside should be yellowish or creamy white. Avoid stark white or greenish colored underside. With cut melons, select red, juicy flesh with black seeds. Keep at room temperature or refrigerate. Peak May to August.

Asparagus. Choose tender, straight green stalks. Avoid spreading or woody stems. Can be stored in plastic bags in the refrigerator crisper for one to three days.

Green Beans. Search for smooth, crisp pods. Avoid limp, wrinkled, or fat overly mature pods. Can be stored in plastic bags in the refrigerator crisper for one to three days.

Broccoli. Look for dark green heads with tightly closed buds. Stalks should be tender yet firm and the leaves should be fresh and unwilted. Avoid yellow buds or rubbery stems.

Can be stored in plastic bags in the refrigerator crisper for two to four days.

Cabbage. Choose heads that are solid and heavy for their size. Avoid heads with splits or yellowed leaves. Can be stored in the crisper for three to seven days.

Carrots. Choose well-shaped, firm, bright orange carrots. Avoid those with splits or blemishes. Can be stored in the crisper for one to four weeks.

Cauliflower. Select firm compact heads with white florets and bright green leaves. Store in the crisper for two to four days.

Celery. Choose celery that has crisp stalks. Leaves should be light or medium green. Avoid limp or yellowed leaves. Can be stored in the crisper for one week.

Mushrooms. Should be firm, white, and relatively clean. Avoid dark bruised ones. Can be stored unwashed, loosely covered on a refrigerator shelf for four days.

Onions. Select onions that do not appear to be ready to sprout. They should be stored in a cool dry place, but not in the refrigerator.

Parsnips. Choose young, straight, firm roots without blemish. Avoid large roots; they tend to be woody. Can be stored unwashed in a perforated bag in the refrigerator for one week.

Bell Peppers. Peppers should be firm and well shaped with shiny flesh. Avoid limp, soft, or wrinkled peppers. Can be stored in the crisper for four to five days.

Potatoes. The best potato for soup is the white or russet potato. They should be stored in a cool dry place away from the sunlight. Most potatoes will keep for two weeks at room temperature.

Scallions. Scallions should have firm white bulbs with crisp green tops. Avoid those with withered or yellow tops. Can be stored in plastic bags in the refrigerator for two to three days.

Shallots. Choose firm, well-shaped bulbs that are heavy for their size. The papery skins should be dry and shiny. Store in a cool dry place. They will keep for several months.

Tomatoes. Should be vine ripened and fully colored. Flavor is best in tomatoes that are stored at room temperature.

Turnips. Choose small, firm, slightly rounded turnips. Avoid large ones as they tend to be strong flavored and woody. Can be stored unwashed in the refrigerator for one week.

Refrigerator and Freezer Storage Times

Use this chart to help make freezing foods a success.

Food	Refrigerator 34–40°F	Freezer 32°F or Lower
Butter	2–4 weeks	6–8 months
Eggs		
Hard cooked	1 week	Do not freeze
Whites (raw)	1 week	12 months
Yolks (raw)	2 days	6 months
Fish		
Lean fish (cod, flounder)	1 day	6 months
Fat fish (salmon, bluefish)	1 day	3 months
Chicken, turkey	1–4 days	6–7 months
Bread		
Quick (baked)	3–7 days	3 months
Yeast (baked)	7–14 days	3 months
Yeast dough	3–5 days	1 month
Fruit		
Apricots, berries, cherries	2–3 days	8–12 months
Melons, nectarines, peaches, plums, pears	3–5 days	8–12 months
Apples, citrus fruits, cranberries	1–2 weeks	8–12 months
Vegetables		
Corn	1 day	8–12 months
Asparagus, green beans	2–3 days	8–12 months
Artichokes, broccoli, collards, lima beans, peas, spinach, turnip greens	3–5 days	8–12 months
Beets, cauliflower, carrots, winter squash	2–3 weeks	8–12 months

Quick Meal Ideas

Grab a bag of combination frozen vegetables and:

■ Add to pasta during the last 3 minutes of cooking time. Drain. Toss with reduced-fat salad dressing and cooked diced chicken for an easy salad.

■ Cook and pile on cooked pizza crusts. Drizzle with reduced-fat salad dressing and top with low-fat mozzarella cheese. Bake to melt the cheese.

■ Stir-fry with cooked chicken or seafood. Add in lite soy sauce. Serve over rice or noodles.

Open some flour tortillas and:

■ Cut into wedges and spray generously with nonstick cooking spray. Bake at 400 degrees until crisp. Sprinkle with dried herbs before baking if desired.

■ Spread reduced-fat cream cheese onto tortillas. Top with thinly sliced meat or vegetables. Roll up, wrap in plastic wrap, and chill. Stick toothpicks into roll 1 inch apart. Cut between the toothpicks for an easy snack or appetizer.

■ Do the same as above, except use 4 tortillas and spread with cream cheese. Add on meat or vegetables and stack the tortillas on each other until all ingredients are used. Cut into wedges to serve.

Use a can of tomatoes and:

■ Drain and toss with hot pasta, herbs, and a dash of Parmesan cheese.

■ Add one 14½-oz can undrained diced tomatoes in place of ½ cup water when preparing instant rice.

■ Add to a slow cooker with chicken recipes in place of 1 cup water.

- Add drained, diced Italian-style tomatoes on top of turkey meatloaf during the last 15 minutes of baking instead of tomato sauce.

- Add ½ cup drained, diced tomatoes to a bowl of hot tomato soup for extra flavor.

Select a bag of frozen corn and:

- Make Quick Succotash. Combine 1 box frozen lima beans with 1 cup frozen corn kernels, a thinly sliced onion, 1 cup milk, and a pinch of honey in a saucepan. Bring to boil and cook on a simmer for 20 minutes until limas are tender and milk is reduced to a few tablespoons. Increase the heat and stir constantly until milk is just glazed over the vegetables.

- Make Easy Corn Chowder. Combine 1 Tbsp olive oil with 1 medium onion in a medium saucepan and cook until onion is golden. Add 2 diced medium potatoes and toss for a few minutes. Add 2 cups fat-free (skim) milk and fresh ground pepper. Simmer for 15 minutes. Add 2 cups frozen corn and return to a simmer.

Buy a carton of eggs or egg substitute and:

- Make Quick Spanish-Style Eggs. Scramble eggs in a nonstick skillet with diced onion and peppers. Pile into a warmed whole-wheat or corn tortilla. Roll up. Top with canned salsa.

- Make Indian-Style Eggs. Add hard-boiled eggs to cooked brown rice. Add a few drops of olive oil and raisins or currants and lightly sautéed chopped apple.

Try a package of dried mushrooms and:

- Toss rehydrated mushrooms with shaped pastas with olive oil and sautéed garlic.

- Fill an omelet with rehydrated mushrooms and bean sprouts and top with a little soy sauce.

- Top any homemade pizza with rehydrated dried mushrooms.

- Rehydrate 1 cup dried mushrooms and sauté in a little olive oil. Add a clove of minced garlic and pile high on 4 pieces of toasted French bread (1 oz each) for a delicious appetizer.

Find a jar of roasted red peppers and:

- Puree 2 roasted peppers with 2 tsp olive oil and 1 tsp capers. Spread on 4 slices of toast for a nice appetizer.

- Toss roasted peppers with pasta and rehydrated sun-dried tomatoes.

- Slice into strips and place on homemade pizzas.

- Toss chopped roasted red peppers into chicken soup.

Take a package of reduced-fat cream cheese and:

- Soften 1 cup cream cheese and mix with 2 Tbsp sugar-free strawberry jam. Spread on 6 slices of whole-grain toast.

- Mix 3 Tbsp into 1 lb of hot mashed potatoes. Add minced chives for extra flavor.

- Spread ⅔ cup of softened cream cheese over 4 slices French bread. Place under the broiler for 2 minutes. Top with slices of ripe tomato and sliced cucumber.

Recipes from the Salad Bar

YEARS AGO WHEN I TAUGHT MY COOKING CLASSES, I was never in favor of using prechopped vegetables. And although I still believe every cook needs to know proper knife skills, I've let up on my staunch belief that everything must be done from scratch. Many of my students only cook for themselves or one other person. Often they lament the point of buying a whole head of broccoli if the recipe only calls for one cup. Too often my students end up wasting vegetables and valuable time.

With today's supermarket salad bar, you can choose from a large variety of items, save time, and avoid waste. There are a few guidelines to follow when choosing ingredients from a salad bar. First, know the store well. Make sure that the salad bar "turns over" several times a day. Ensure that there are sneeze guards installed. Check that cold foods are cold and hot foods are hot. Inspect the vegetables and make sure there are no signs of wilting, browning, or unpleasant odors.

In the following recipes, if some of the items are not available from your salad bar, simply buy them from the produce department and prepare them according to what the recipe calls for.

*R*ecipes

Salad Bar Stir-Fry

Serves 4 **Serving size: 1 cup tofu, 1/2 cup vegetables**
Preparation time: 15 minutes
Cooking time: 15 minutes

SALAD BAR: tofu, onions, peppers, carrots, broccoli

ALSO VISIT: shelves for broth, soy sauce, oil, red pepper flakes, arrowroot powder

2	tsp canola or peanut oil
1	lb extra-firm tofu, cubed
1	tsp cornstarch or arrowroot powder
1	clove garlic, minced
1/2	cup minced onion
1/2	cup shredded carrot
1/2	cup sliced green or red bell pepper
1/2	cup broccoli florets
1/2	cup low-fat, low-sodium chicken broth
1	Tbsp lite soy sauce
1	tsp sesame oil
	Dash crushed red pepper flakes

1. Coat the tofu with the cornstarch. In a nonstick wok, heat the oil over high heat. Lower the heat to medium-high and stir-fry the tofu cubes until golden brown, about 5–7 minutes. Remove tofu from wok and place on paper towels.

2. In the same wok, add the garlic and onion and stir-fry for 1 minute. Add the carrots and stir-fry for 3 minutes. Add the peppers and stir-fry for 3 minutes. Add the broccoli and broth. Cover and steam for 3–4 minutes, until broccoli is bright green and crunchy. Return the tofu to the wok.

3. Mix together the remaining ingredients. Toss with vegetables and tofu and serve.

Exchanges

1 Vegetable
1 Meat
1/2 Fat

Calories 121
   Calories from Fat . . 52
Total Fat . . . . 6 g
   Saturated Fat . . . . . . 1 g
Cholesterol . . . . 0 mg
Sodium . . . . 308 mg
Carbohydrate . . . . 9 g
   Dietary Fiber . . . . . . 2 g
   Sugars . . . . 6 g
Protein . . . . 10 g

Asian Coleslaw

Serves 4   Serving size: 1/2 cup
Preparation time: 10 minutes

SALAD BAR: shredded cabbage

ALSO VISIT: shelves for vinegar, soy sauce, sesame oil, spices, honey

2 cups shredded cabbage (or coleslaw mix from produce department)

Dressing:
1/3 cup rice vinegar

2 Tbsp lite soy sauce

2 tsp sesame oil

1 tsp ground ginger

2 tsp honey

1. Place the cabbage in a salad bowl.

2. Combine the remaining ingredients in a blender. Pour over the cabbage and mix well.

Exchanges
1 Vegetable
1/2 Fat

Calories	46
Calories from Fat	. . 21
Total Fat	2 g
Saturated Fat	1 g
Cholesterol	0 mg
Sodium	309 mg
Carbohydrate	7 g
Dietary Fiber	1 g
Sugars	5 g
Protein	1 g

Spicy Summer Gazpacho

Serves 6 **Serving size: 1-1/4 cups**
Preparation time: 5 minutes
Standing time: 2 hours

SALAD BAR: cucumbers, tomatoes, green pepper, onion

ALSO VISIT: shelves for tomato juice, vinegar, hot sauce

1	cup sliced cucumbers
2	cups chopped tomatoes
1/2	cup sliced green pepper
1/2	cup sliced onion
4	cups spicy tomato juice (or regular tomato juice if you wish)
1/3	cup red wine vinegar
1/4	tsp hot sauce (optional)
	Fresh ground pepper and salt to taste

1. In a blender, puree half of the vegetables with half of the tomato juice.

2. Pour the puree into a bowl, and add the remaining tomato juice, red wine vinegar, hot sauce, and salt and pepper.

3. Add the remaining chopped vegetables. Refrigerate for 2 hours.

Exchanges

2 Vegetable

Calories 53
Calories from Fat . . . 4
Total Fat . . . . 0 g
Saturated Fat . . . . . . 0 g
Cholesterol . . . . 0 mg
Sodium . . . . 593 mg
Carbohydrate . . . . . . 13 g
Dietary Fiber . . . . . . 2 g
Sugars . . . . 9 g
Protein . . . . 2 g

Indian Lentils

Serves 4   Serving size: 1/2 cup
Preparation time: 15 minutes
Cooking time: 10 minutes

SALAD BAR: lentils, tomatoes, green pepper, onion, green onion

ALSO VISIT: shelves for spices, vinegar, oil, canned lentils if necessary

2	tsp canola oil
1	tsp fresh minced ginger
1/2	cup minced onion
1/4	cup chopped green pepper
1/2	tsp coriander
1/4	tsp turmeric
1/4	tsp chili powder
1/2	cup diced tomatoes
2	cups cooked lentils
1	Tbsp white wine vinegar

Garnish: 2 Tbsp minced green onion

1. In a heavy skillet over medium-high heat, heat the oil. Add the ginger and onion and sauté for 2 minutes. Add the green pepper and sauté for 2 minutes, stirring occasionally. Add the coriander, turmeric, and chili powder and coat the vegetables well.

2. Add the tomatoes and cook for 2 minutes. Add the lentils and cook for 2 minutes. Add the vinegar and cook for 1 minute more. Garnish with green onions and serve.

Exchanges

1 Starch
1 Vegetable
1 Very Lean Meat

Calories 128	
Calories from Fat . . 25	
Total Fat . . . . 3 g	
Saturated Fat . . . . . . 0 g	
Cholesterol . . . . 0 mg	
Sodium . . . . 51 mg	
Carbohydrate . . . . . . 19 g	
Dietary Fiber . . . . . . 7 g	
Sugars . . . . 4 g	
Protein . . . . 8 g	

Moroccan Carrot Salad

Serves 4   Serving size: 1/2 cup carrots, 1/2 cup watercress
Preparation time: 10 minutes

SALAD BAR: carrots, olives, watercress

ALSO VISIT: shelves for orange flower water, cinnamon, honey

> 2   cups shredded carrot
> 1/3 cup sliced green olives
> 1   small orange, peeled, sliced, and segmented
> 3   Tbsp orange juice
> 1   Tbsp lemon juice
> 2   tsp orange flower water
> 1/2 tsp cinnamon
> 1   Tbsp honey
> 2   cups watercress

1. In a medium bowl, combine the carrots, olives, and orange.

2. Whisk together the remaining ingredients except the watercress. Add to the salad and toss.

3. Line individual plates with the watercress. Top with carrot salad.

Exchanges

1/2 Fruit
1 Vegetable
1/2 Monounsaturated Fat

Calories 78
    Calories from Fat . . 12
Total Fat . . . . 1 g
    Saturated Fat . . . . . . 0 g
Cholesterol . . . . 0 mg
Sodium . . . . 125 mg
Carbohydrate . . . . . . 17 g
    Dietary Fiber . . . . . . 3 g
    Sugars . . . . 12 g
Protein . . . . 2 g

Cauliflower, Pea, and Chickpea Curry

Serves 4   Serving size: 1 cup
Preparation time: 10 minutes
Cooking time: 10 minutes

SALAD BAR: cauliflower, peas, chickpeas, onion, tomato, raisins

ALSO VISIT: shelves for coconut milk, spices, flour

> 2 tsp canola oil
>
> 1/2 cup diced onion
>
> 2 tsp curry powder
>
> 2 cups cauliflower florets
>
> 1/2 cup low-fat, low-sodium chicken broth
>
> 1 cup cooked peas
>
> 1/2 cup cooked chickpeas
>
> 1 Tbsp unbleached white flour
>
> 1 14-oz can lite coconut milk (or use 1 can evaporated skim milk with 1 tsp coconut extract added)
>
> 2 tsp sugar
>
> 1/4 cup diced tomato
>
> Fresh ground pepper and salt to taste

Garnish: 2 Tbsp raisins

1. Heat the oil in a heavy skillet over medium-high heat. Add the onion and sauté for 2 minutes. Add the curry powder and sauté for 1 minute.

2. Add the cauliflower and broth. Cover and steam for 3 minutes, until cauliflower is softened but still crisp. Add the peas and chickpeas. Sprinkle the vegetables with the flour. Sauté for 2 minutes.

3. Mix together the coconut milk and sugar. Add to the vegetables. Cook for 2 minutes. Add the tomatoes and cook for 1 minute. Season to taste. Garnish with raisins and serve.

With Lite Coconut Milk Exchanges

1 1/2 Carbohydrate
1 1/2 Fat

Calories 184
   Calories from Fat . . 73
Total Fat . . . . 8 g
   Saturated Fat . . . . . . 3 g
Cholesterol . . . . 0 mg
Sodium . . . . 150 mg
Carbohydrate . . . . . . 25 g
   Dietary Fiber . . . . . . 5 g
   Sugars . . . . 12 g
Protein . . . . 5 g

With Evaporated Skim Milk Exchanges

1 Skim Milk
1 Carbohydrate
1 Monounsaturated Fat

Calories 197
   Calories from Fat . . 30
Total Fat . . . . 3 g
   Saturated Fat . . . . . . 0 g
Cholesterol . . . . 3 mg
Sodium . . . . 219 mg
Carbohydrate . . . . . . 32 g
   Dietary Fiber . . . . . . 5 g
   Sugars . . . . 18 g
Protein . . . . 12 g

Zucchini and Yellow Squash Puttanesca

Serves 4   Serving size: 1/2 cup
Preparation time: 10 minutes
Cooking time: 15 minutes

SALAD BAR: onion, zucchini, yellow squash
ALSO VISIT: shelves for marinara sauce, anchovies, olives, capers

1	tsp olive oil
1/2	cup diced onion
1	cup sliced zucchini
1	cup sliced yellow squash
1	cup marinara sauce
2	anchovies, mashed, or 2 tsp anchovy paste
1/3	cup oil-cured olives, pitted, rinsed, and drained
2	tsp capers
	Fresh ground pepper to taste

1. In a skillet over medium-high heat, heat the oil. Add the onion and sauté for 3 minutes. Add the zucchini and yellow squash and sauté for 5 minutes, stirring occasionally.

2. Add the marinara sauce, lower the heat, and simmer for 3 minutes. Add the anchovies, olives, and capers and simmer for 4 minutes. Add pepper to taste.

Exchanges
2 Vegetable
1 Monounsaturated Fat

Calories 89
  Calories from Fat . . 45
Total Fat . . . . 5 g
  Saturated Fat . . . . . . 1 g
Cholesterol . . . . 4 mg
Sodium . . . . 486 mg
Carbohydrate . . . . 4 g
  Dietary Fiber . . . . . . 4 g
  Sugars . . . . 5 g
Protein . . . . 3 g

Cantaloupe, Chicken, and Mango Chutney Salad

Serves 4   Serving size: 3 oz chicken, 1/2 cup fruit
Preparation time: 15 minutes
Cooking time: 10 minutes
Chilling time: 1 hour

SALAD BAR: melon, celery, green onions, raisins

ALSO VISIT: poultry case for chicken; shelves for broth, mayonnaise, chutney, spices

1	lb chicken breast tenderloins
1/4	cup low-fat, low-sodium chicken broth
2	cups cut-up cantaloupe or honeydew melon
1	cup sliced celery
1/4	cup sliced green onions
2	Tbsp raisins
1/2	cup low-fat mayonnaise
2	Tbsp reduced-fat sour cream
1/4	cup mango chutney
1/4	tsp ground ginger
1/4	tsp cinnamon

1. Place the chicken tenderloins on a broiler pan. Sprinkle with the chicken broth. Broil for about 2–3 minutes per side until chicken is cooked through.

2. Cut the tenderloins in half. In a large bowl, combine the tenderloins with the melon, celery, green onions, and raisins.

3. In a small bowl combine the mayonnaise, sour cream, chutney, ginger, and cinnamon. Mix well. Combine the dressing with the salad. Refrigerate for 1 hour.

Exchanges
2 1/2 Carbohydrate
3 Very Lean Meat

Calories 301
   Calories from Fat . . 51
Total Fat . . . . 6 g
   Saturated Fat . . . . . . 1 g
Cholesterol . . . . 71 mg
Sodium . . . . 587 mg
Carbohydrate . . . . . . 34 g
   Dietary Fiber . . . . . . 2 g
   Sugars . . . . 25 g
Protein . . . . 27 g

Roasted Cherry Tomato and Bell Pepper Pasta

Serves 4   Serving size: 1/2 cup pasta, 1/2 cup vegetables
Preparation time: 15 minutes   Cooking time: 35 minutes

SALAD BAR: cherry tomatoes, green onions, peppers, olives

ALSO VISIT: shelves for pasta, spices, anchovy paste; produce section for garlic; dairy section for Parmesan cheese

- 1 lb cherry tomatoes
- 3 tsp olive oil, divided
- 3 garlic cloves, sliced
- 1 cup sliced bell pepper (red or green)
- 1 tsp anchovy paste
- 1/4 cup sliced green onions
- 1 tsp dried oregano
- 1/4 tsp salt
- 1/2 tsp black pepper
- 1/2 cup pitted black olives
- 2 cups cooked angel hair pasta
- 1/4 cup freshly grated Parmesan cheese

Exchanges
1 1/2 Starch
2 Vegetable
1 Monounsaturated Fat

Calories 213
  Calories from Fat . . 69
Total Fat . . . . 8 g
  Saturated Fat . . . . . . 2 g
Cholesterol . . . . 6 mg
Sodium . . . . 458 mg
Carbohydrate . . . . . . 32 g
  Dietary Fiber . . . . . . 4 g
  Sugars . . . . 6 g
Protein . . . . 8 g

1. Preheat oven to 400°F. Place cherry tomatoes, 2 tsp oil, and garlic in a baking pan sprayed with nonstick cooking spray. Roast uncovered for 20–25 minutes until tomatoes are soft and slightly browned. Remove from oven and set aside.

2. Prepare pasta according to package directions. Meanwhile, in a skillet over medium-high heat, heat remaining 1 tsp oil. Add peppers and sauté for 3–4 minutes, stirring occasionally. Reduce heat to medium. Add green onions and anchovy paste and sauté for 2 minutes more. Add seasonings and olives. Cook 1 minute more. Add roasted tomatoes to the peppers and mix well. Toss tomato and pepper mixture with pasta, and top each serving with cheese.

Pan-Seared Chicken with Cherry Tomato Salsa

Serves 4   Serving size: 3 oz chicken, 1/2 cup salsa
Preparation time: 10 minutes
Cooking time: 15 minutes

SALAD BAR: cherry tomatoes, red onion, red bell pepper

ALSO VISIT: poultry case for chicken; produce section for cilantro, garlic; shelves for lime juice, olive oil

1	lb boneless, skinless chicken breast halves
1	Tbsp garlic-flavored olive oil (or plain olive oil)
16	cherry tomatoes, halved
1/2	cup sliced red onion
1/2	cup diced red bell pepper
1	jalapeño pepper, minced
2	Tbsp minced cilantro
2	garlic cloves, minced
1/4	cup lime juice
1/4	tsp salt
1/2	tsp black pepper

1. Brush each chicken breast with olive oil. In a nonstick skillet over medium heat, cook the chicken for about 4–6 minutes per side until golden brown and no longer pink inside. Remove from the skillet and keep warm.

2. Combine the remaining ingredients in a small bowl and serve with the chicken.

Exchanges
3 Vegetable
3 Very Lean Meat
1 Monounsaturated Fat

Calories 204
  Calories from Fat . . 59
Total Fat . . . . 7 g
  Saturated Fat . . . . . . 2 g
Cholesterol . . . . 68 mg
Sodium . . . . 214 mg
Carbohydrate . . . . 9 g
  Dietary Fiber . . . . . . 2 g
  Sugars . . . . 5 g
Protein . . . . 27 g

Everything from the Garden Frittata

Serves 4   Serving size: 2 eggs, 1/2 cup vegetables
Preparation time: 15 minutes   Cooking time: 20 minutes

SALAD BAR: onion, peppers, zucchini, broccoli, tomatoes

ALSO VISIT: dairy section for eggs and Parmesan cheese; shelves for spices

2	tsp olive oil
1/2	cup chopped onion
2	garlic cloves, minced
1/2	cup diced red bell pepper
1/2	cup diced green bell pepper
1/2	cup diced zucchini
1/2	cup chopped broccoli
8	eggs, beaten
2	Tbsp water
1/2	tsp dried oregano
1/2	tsp dried basil
	Fresh ground pepper and salt to taste
2	tomatoes, thinly sliced
3	Tbsp Parmesan cheese

Exchanges

2 Vegetable
2 Medium-Fat Meat
1 Fat

Calories 237
  Calories from Fat . 129
Total Fat . . . . 14 g
  Saturated Fat . . . . . . 6 g
Cholesterol . . . . 432 mg
Sodium . . . . 235 mg
Carbohydrate . . . . . . 11 g
  Dietary Fiber . . . . . . 3 g
  Sugars . . . . 7 g
Protein . . . . 17 g

1. Heat oil in a large nonstick, oven-safe skillet over medium heat. Add onion and garlic and sauté for 3 minutes. Add peppers, zucchini, and broccoli and sauté for 4 minutes.

2. Combine eggs, water, and dry seasonings in a bowl. Pour mixture over vegetables in the skillet and cook over medium heat for about 8 minutes, until eggs look almost set on the bottom. Arrange tomatoes in circles on top of eggs and sprinkle with cheese.

3. Set oven to broil. Place skillet in oven and broil 7 inches from the heat until eggs are set on top and cheese is lightly browned. Watch carefully. Cut into wedges to serve.

Hot Pita Pocket Italiano

**Serves 4 Serving size: 1 pita bread, 1 cup vegetables,
2 Tbsp cheese**
Preparation time: 15 minutes
Cooking time: 17 minutes

SALAD BAR: onion, zucchini, yellow squash, broccoli, carrots, cherry
tomatoes

ALSO VISIT: shelves for marinara sauce, spices; dairy section for cheese;
bakery section for pita

2	tsp olive oil
1/2	cup diced onion
1	cup diced zucchini
1/2	cup diced yellow squash
1/2	cup chopped broccoli
1/2	cup sliced carrots
1/2	cup halved cherry tomatoes
1	cup marinara sauce
1	tsp dried oregano
1/2	tsp dried basil
1/2	cup shredded low-fat mozzarella cheese
4	1-oz whole-wheat mini pita breads, cut open to form a pocket

1. Preheat the oven to 400°F. Heat the oil in a skillet over medium heat. Add the onion and zucchini and sauté for 5 minutes. Add the yellow squash, broccoli, and carrots and sauté for 4 minutes. Add the cherry tomatoes and sauté for 2 minutes.

2. Meanwhile, add the dried seasonings to the marinara sauce and stir.

3. Divide the vegetable mixture among the four pita breads. Top with sauce and sprinkle with cheese.

4. Place the pita breads upright against each other in a small casserole dish. Bake for 5–6 minutes until hot and cheese has melted.

Exchanges
1 1/2 Starch
2 Vegetable
1 Monounsaturated Fat

Calories 206
 Calories from Fat . . 64
Total Fat . . . . 7 g
 Saturated Fat . . . . . . 2 g
Cholesterol . . . . 10 mg
Sodium . . . . 448 mg
Carbohydrate . . . . . . 28 g
 Dietary Fiber . . . . . . 6 g
 Sugars . . . . 8 g
Protein . . . . 10 g

Mediterranean Pizzas

Serves 4   Serving size: 1 pita, 1 oz cheese, 1/2 cup chickpea spread
Preparation time: 15 minutes
Cooking time: 5 minutes

SALAD BAR: chickpeas, feta cheese, tomatoes, olives

ALSO VISIT: shelves for spices, tahini (sesame paste); bakery section for pita

2	cups chickpeas, rinsed and drained
3	cloves garlic
2	Tbsp lemon juice
1	tsp cumin
2	tsp olive oil
2	Tbsp tahini
1	cup crumbled feta cheese
1/2	cup diced tomatoes
1/2	cup sliced black olives
1	tsp Italian seasoning
4	6-inch whole-wheat pita breads

1. Preheat the oven to 425°F. In a blender, combine the chickpeas, garlic, lemon juice, cumin, olive oil, and tahini and puree until smooth. (You may need to start by blending half of the chickpeas with the liquid before adding the rest. If the mixture is too thick to blend, add a small amount of warm water or juice from the chickpeas.) Set aside.

2. Spread some of the chickpea puree on each pita and arrange on a baking sheet. Top with feta cheese, tomatoes, olives, and Italian seasoning.

3. Bake at 425°F for 5 minutes until cheese is lightly browned.

Exchanges
4 Starch
1 Very Lean Meat
2 Fat

Calories 443
  Calories from Fat . 158
Total Fat . . . . 18 g
  Saturated Fat . . . . . . 5 g
Cholesterol . . . . 25 mg
Sodium . . . . 609 mg
Carbohydrate . . . . . . 59 g
  Dietary Fiber . . . . . 10 g
  Sugars . . . . 9 g
Protein . . . . 19 g

Fusilli with Spinach-Broccoli Pesto

Serves 4   Serving size: 1 cup
Preparation time: 15 minutes
Cooking time: 15 minutes (includes cooking pasta)

SALAD BAR: broccoli, spinach

ALSO VISIT: shelves for oil, broth, pasta; produce section for parsley; dairy section for Parmesan cheese

2 cups broccoli florets

2 cups loosely packed fresh spinach

1/2 cup Italian parsley

3 green onions, minced

3 cloves garlic, minced

1/4 cup grated Parmesan cheese

1/4 cup low-fat, low-sodium chicken broth

2 Tbsp olive oil

1 Tbsp fresh lemon juice

1/4 tsp fresh ground pepper

1/4 tsp salt

4 cups cooked fusilli noodles, hot

1. In a steamer over boiling water, steam the broccoli florets for about 4 minutes or until tender. Drain.

2. Combine the cooked broccoli with the spinach, parsley, green onions, garlic, Parmesan cheese, broth, olive oil, lemon juice, pepper, and salt in a food processor or blender and process until smooth.

3. Toss the pesto with the cooked fusilli.

Exchanges

3 Starch
1 Vegetable
1 1/2 Monounsaturated Fat

Calories 325
 Calories from Fat . . 94
Total Fat . . . . 10 g
 Saturated Fat . . . . . . 3 g
Cholesterol . . . . 8 mg
Sodium . . . . 352 mg
Carbohydrate . . . . . . 51 g
 Dietary Fiber . . . . . . 6 g
 Sugars . . . . 4 g
Protein . . . . 13 g

Greek Chicken Gyros

Serves 4   Serving size: 1 pita, 3 oz chicken, 1/4 cup feta cheese
Preparation time: 15 minutes
Cooking time: 20 minutes

SALAD BAR: cucumber, tomato, spinach, feta cheese

ALSO VISIT: bakery section for pita; dairy section for yogurt; poultry case for chicken; produce section for dill

- 4 6-oz whole-wheat pita breads
- 2 tsp olive oil
- 1 large onion, thinly sliced
- 1 lb boneless, skinless chicken breasts, cut into very thin strips
- 1/2 cup plain nonfat yogurt
- 1/2 cup chopped cucumber
- 2 Tbsp minced fresh dill
- 1/2 cup torn spinach leaves
- 1/2 cup chopped tomatoes
- 1 cup crumbled feta cheese

1. Wrap the pita breads in aluminum foil and heat at 400°F for about 10 minutes. Lower the oven temperature and keep warm.

2. Heat the oil in a skillet over medium-high heat. Add the onion and chicken and sauté for 5–6 minutes until onion is browned and chicken is cooked through.

3. Combine the cucumbers, yogurt, and dill. Set aside.

4. Remove the pitas from the oven. Arrange the onion and chicken mixture over each pita. Top with spinach, tomatoes, and feta cheese. Fold pita sides in to form a cone. Wrap the bottom of each cone with foil. Serve with the cucumber-yogurt sauce.

Exchanges

2 Starch
1 Vegetable
4 Lean Meat

Calories 410
  Calories from Fat . 114
Total Fat . . . . 13 g
  Saturated Fat . . . . . . 5 g
Cholesterol . . . . 94 mg
Sodium . . . . 537 mg
Carbohydrate . . . . . . 39 g
  Dietary Fiber . . . . . . 3 g
  Sugars . . . . 9 g
Protein . . . . 37 g

Spinach Fettuccine Primavera

Serves 4   Serving size: 1 cup linguine and vegetables
Preparation time: 15 minutes
Cooking time: 15 minutes

SALAD BAR: onion, zucchini, broccoli, carrots, tomatoes

ALSO VISIT: produce section for basil; shelves for pasta, spices; dairy section for cheese

2	tsp olive oil
1	cup diced onion
1 1/2	cups sliced zucchini
1	cup broccoli florets
1	cup sliced carrots
2	cups diced tomatoes
2	Tbsp minced fresh basil
1	tsp sugar
1/4	tsp salt
1/2	tsp fresh ground pepper
4	cups cooked spinach linguine, hot
1/2	cup grated Parmesan cheese

1. Heat the oil in a skillet over medium-high heat. Add the onion and sauté for 2–4 minutes, stirring occasionally. Reduce the heat to medium. Add the zucchini, broccoli, carrots, and tomatoes and sauté for 5 minutes. Add the basil. Bring to a boil, then lower the heat and simmer for 5 minutes. Add the sugar, salt, and pepper and cook 1 minute more.

2. Toss the vegetables with the pasta. Top each serving with cheese.

Exchanges
3 Starch
3 Vegetable
1 Fat

Calories 438
  Calories from Fat . . 75
Total Fat . . . . 8 g
  Saturated Fat . . . . . . 4 g
Cholesterol . . . . 15 mg
Sodium . . . . 446 mg
Carbohydrate . . . . . . 60 g
  Dietary Fiber . . . . . . 7 g
  Sugars . . . . 11 g
Protein . . . . 16 g

Shrimp Provençal

Serves 4   Serving size: 4 oz shrimp, 1/2 cup vegetables
Preparation time: 15 minutes
Cooking time: 12 minutes

SALAD BAR: mushrooms, green onions, zucchini, tomatoes

ALSO VISIT: frozen-food section for shrimp; shelves for lemon juice, spices

1 lb cooked medium shrimp, peeled and deveined (Tip: Buy already cooked frozen shrimp, rinse with water, and pat dry before use.)

1 Tbsp lemon juice

1 Tbsp olive oil

1 cup sliced mushrooms

1/2 cup sliced green onions

1/2 cup sliced zucchini

2 Tbsp minced parsley

1/2 tsp dried oregano

2 cups halved cherry tomatoes or 2 cups diced tomatoes

2 Tbsp dry white wine (optional)

1/4 tsp salt

1/2 tsp fresh ground pepper

Pinch crushed red pepper

Garnish: oregano or parsley sprigs

1. Combine the shrimp and lemon juice and set aside.

2. Heat the oil in a skillet over medium-high heat. Add the mushrooms, green onions, and zucchini and sauté for 5 minutes. Add the parsley and oregano. Add the tomatoes, wine, salt, pepper, and crushed red pepper. Simmer for 5 minutes.

3. Add the shrimp and simmer for 2 more minutes. Garnish with sprigs of oregano or parsley and serve.

Exchanges
2 Vegetable
3 Very Lean Meat
1/2 Monounsaturated Fat

Calories 177
  Calories from Fat . . 46
Total Fat . . . . 5 g
  Saturated Fat . . . . . . 1 g
Cholesterol . . . . 220 mg
Sodium . . . . 411 mg
Carbohydrate . . . . 8 g
  Dietary Fiber . . . . . . 2 g
  Sugars . . . . 4 g
Protein . . . . 25 g

Vegetable, Turkey, and Lamb Burgers

Serves 4   Serving size: 4 oz (1/4 recipe)
Preparation time: 15 minutes
Cooking time: 15 minutes

SALAD BAR: onion, carrot, celery, zucchini

ALSO VISIT: meat case for lamb, turkey; produce section for mint; shelves for spices, Worcestershire sauce; dairy section for Parmesan cheese

2	tsp olive oil
1/2	cup finely diced onion
1/2	cup finely diced carrot
1/2	cup finely sliced celery
1/2	cup finely sliced zucchini
1/2	lb ground turkey breast
1/2	lb lean ground lamb
3	Tbsp grated Parmesan cheese
1	Tbsp Worcestershire sauce
1	tsp minced fresh mint
1/4	tsp salt
1/2	tsp fresh ground black pepper

1. Preheat the broiler or an outdoor grill.

2. Heat the oil in a skillet over medium-high heat. Add the onion, carrots, celery, and zucchini and sauté for 5 minutes, stirring occasionally.

3. In a medium bowl, combine the sautéed vegetables with the remaining ingredients. Gently form into patties.

4. Broil or grill patties 4 inches from the heat source for about 6–9 minutes per side.

Exchanges
1 Vegetable
3 Lean Meat
1/2 Monounsaturated Fat

Calories	214
Calories from Fat	93
Total Fat	10 g
Saturated Fat	4 g
Cholesterol	72 mg
Sodium	265 mg
Carbohydrate	6 g
Dietary Fiber	1 g
Sugars	3 g
Protein	23 g

Halibut En Papillote

Serves 4   Serving size: 3–4 oz fish, 3/4 cup vegetables
Preparation time: 10 minutes
Cooking time: 10 minutes

SALAD BAR: onion, carrots, celery, tomato

ALSO VISIT: seafood section for halibut; produce section for tarragon; shelves for white wine, spices

1	lb halibut fillets (1 inch thick)
2	tsp olive oil
1	cup diced onion
1	cup sliced carrots
1/2	cup sliced celery
1	cup diced tomato
1/2	cup dry white wine
2	tsp minced fresh tarragon
1/4	tsp salt
1/2	tsp fresh ground black pepper
	Dash crushed red pepper

1. Preheat the oven to 425°F.

2. Tear off four large squares of aluminum foil. Place a halibut fillet on the center of each square. Drizzle with some of the olive oil. Sprinkle each fillet evenly with onion, carrot, celery, and tomato. Drizzle with white wine. Sprinkle with tarragon, salt, pepper, and crushed red pepper.

3. Fold each square into a packet and place all four packets on a baking sheet. Bake for 10 minutes. Remove the packets from the oven and let cool slightly before serving.

Exchanges

2 Vegetable
3 Very Lean Meat
1/2 Monounsaturated Fat

Calories 192
    Calories from Fat . . 45
Total Fat . . . . 5 g
    Saturated Fat . . . . . . 1 g
Cholesterol . . . . 36 mg
Sodium . . . . 235 mg
Carbohydrate . . . . 9 g
    Dietary Fiber . . . . . . 2 g
    Sugars . . . . 6 g
Protein . . . . 25 g

Spiced Chicken Cutlets

Serves 4   Serving size: 4 oz (3–4 oz chicken and vegetable sauce)
Preparation time: 15 minutes
Cooking time: 20 minutes

SALAD BAR: green onions, peppers, carrots, cauliflower

ALSO VISIT: shelves for spices, broth, brown sugar, raisins; meat department for chicken

2	tsp olive oil
1/2	cup sliced green onions
1	cup sliced red or green bell pepper
1/2	cup sliced carrots
1/2	cup cauliflower florets
1 1/2	cups low-fat, low-sodium chicken broth
1/4	tsp turmeric
1	Tbsp dark brown sugar
1	tsp cinnamon
1	tsp allspice
1	tsp cumin
	Pinch crushed red pepper
1/4	tsp coriander
1	lb chicken cutlets
1/4	cup raisins

1. In a skillet over medium-high heat, heat the oil. Add the green onions, bell peppers, carrots, and cauliflower and sauté for 7 minutes, stirring occasionally. Add the broth and turmeric and bring to a boil. Lower the heat and simmer for 5 minutes.

2. Combine the brown sugar, cinnamon, allspice, cumin, crushed red pepper, and coriander. Rub mixture onto the surface of the chicken cutlets.

3. Add the chicken to the simmering vegetables and cook covered for 6–7 minutes. Add the raisins and cook for 1 minute more.

Exchanges
1 Carbohydrate
4 Very Lean Meat

Calories 213
 Calories from Fat . . 37
Total Fat . . . . 4 g
 Saturated Fat . . . . . . 1 g
Cholesterol . . . . 64 mg
Sodium . . . . 323 mg
Carbohydrate . . . . . . 16 g
 Dietary Fiber . . . . . . 2 g
 Sugars . . . . 12 g
Protein . . . . 28 g

Chilled Cucumber and Watercress Soup

Serves 4   Serving size: 1 cup
Preparation time: 5 minutes
Standing time: 2–4 hours

SALAD BAR: watercress, cucumbers, onion

ALSO VISIT: dairy section for sour cream, milk; shelves for bottled lemon juice, spices

1 1/2	cups fat-free sour cream
1/2	cup low-fat milk
1/2	cup washed watercress sprigs
2	cups diced cucumbers
1	Tbsp lemon juice
1/4	cup chopped onion
1/4	tsp salt
1/2	tsp fresh ground black pepper

Garnish: 1/2 cup fat-free sour cream; watercress sprigs

1. Combine the sour cream, milk, watercress, cucumbers, lemon juice, onion, salt, and pepper in a blender. Blend until smooth.

2. Chill the soup in the refrigerator for 2–4 hours. Divide into bowls and garnish with sour cream and watercress sprigs before serving.

Exchanges
1 1/2 Carbohydrate

Calories	129
Calories from Fat	4
Total Fat	0 g
Saturated Fat	0 g
Cholesterol	9 mg
Sodium	309 mg
Carbohydrate	24 g
Dietary Fiber	1 g
Sugars	11 g
Protein	6 g

Summer Fruit Soup

Serves 4   Serving size: 1 cup
Preparation time: 5 minutes
Standing time: 1–2 hours

SALAD BAR: melon, strawberries

ALSO VISIT: dairy section for yogurt; refrigerated section for orange juice; shelves for bottled lemon juice, spices

3	cups cut cantaloupe or honeydew melon
1	cup sliced strawberries
1/2	cup plain fat-free yogurt
1/2	cup orange juice
1/4	cup lemon juice
2	tsp minced crystallized ginger or 1/2 tsp ground ginger
2	Tbsp sugar

Garnish: 1/2 cup reduced-fat sour cream; mint sprigs

1. Combine all ingredients and chill for 1–2 hours. Garnish with a dollop of low-fat sour cream and a mint sprig.

Exchanges
2 Carbohydrate

Calories 150
   Calories from Fat . . 27
Total Fat . . . . 3 g
   Saturated Fat . . . . . . 1 g
Cholesterol . . . . 1 mg
Sodium . . . . 58 mg
Carbohydrate . . . . . . 29 g
   Dietary Fiber . . . . . . 2 g
   Sugars . . . . 25 g
Protein . . . . 5 g

Spanish Vegetable Paella

Serves 6   Serving size: 1 cup rice, 1/2 cup vegetables
Preparation time: 15 minutes
Cooking time: 35 minutes

SALAD BAR: peppers, zucchini, yellow squash, carrots, tomatoes
ALSO VISIT: shelves for rice, broth, spices

2	tsp olive oil
1	cup diced onion
2	cups sliced green or red bell peppers
1	cup sliced zucchini
1/2	cup sliced yellow squash
1/2	cup sliced carrots
2	cups diced tomatoes
2	cups long-grain rice
3 1/2	cups low-fat, low-sodium chicken broth
	Pinch saffron threads
	Fresh ground pepper and salt to taste

1. In a large stockpot or Dutch oven over medium-high heat, heat the oil. Add the onion, peppers, zucchini, and yellow squash and sauté for 5 minutes. Add the carrots and tomatoes and sauté for 5 minutes more.

2. Add the rice and sauté for 3 minutes. Add the broth and saffron and bring to a boil. Lower the heat, cover, and simmer for 20 minutes until rice is tender and has absorbed the broth. Add salt and pepper to taste.

Exchanges
3 Starch
2 Vegetable

Calories 290
  Calories from Fat . . 21
Total Fat . . . . 2 g
  Saturated Fat . . . . . . 0 g
Cholesterol . . . . 0 mg
Sodium . . . . 294 mg
Carbohydrate . . . . . . 59 g
  Dietary Fiber . . . . . . 3 g
  Sugars . . . . 5 g
Protein . . . . 8 g

Low-Fat Dinner Burritos

Serves 4   Serving size: 1 burrito (1/2 cup beans, 1/2 cup vegetables, 2 Tbsp cheese, 2 Tbsp salsa, 1 10-inch tortilla)
Preparation time: 15 minutes   Cooking time: 17 minutes

SALAD BAR: kidney beans, onion, peppers, zucchini, carrot

ALSO VISIT: dairy for cheese, tortillas; shelves for salsa, spices

> 2 cups kidney beans
>
> 2 tsp canola oil, divided
>
> 1/2 cup sliced onion
>
> 2 tsp chili powder
>
> 1 cup red bell pepper strips
>
> 1 cup sliced zucchini
>
> 1 cup sliced or shredded carrot
>
> 1/4 tsp cumin
>
> Fresh ground pepper and salt to taste
>
> 1/2 cup low-fat cheddar or Monterey Jack cheese
>
> 4 10-inch whole-wheat tortillas, warmed in the oven for 5 minutes
>
> 1/2 cup store-bought salsa

1. In a bowl, mash beans coarsely with a potato masher.

2. In a skillet over medium-high heat, heat 1 tsp oil. Add beans and onions and sauté for 6 minutes. Turn heat to high and sauté for another 3 minutes. Remove bean mixture from skillet and set aside, but keep warm.

3. Lower heat to medium-high and add remaining 1 tsp oil to skillet. Add peppers, zucchini, and carrot. Sauté for 5 minutes. Add cumin, pepper, and salt and sauté for 2 minutes, stirring occasionally.

4. Spread 1/4 bean mixture onto a warmed tortilla. Top with vegetables. Sprinkle with cheese. Fold over sides and roll up. Serve with salsa.

Exchanges
4 Starch
1 Vegetable
1 Lean Meat

Calories 393
  Calories from Fat . . 81
Total Fat . . . . 9 g
  Saturated Fat . . . . . . 2 g
Cholesterol . . . . 3 mg
Sodium . . . . 896 mg
Carbohydrate . . . . . . 62 g
  Dietary Fiber . . . . . 10 g
  Sugars . . . . 10 g
Protein . . . . 18 g

Summer Main Dish Pasta Salad

Serves 4   **Serving size: 1 cup pasta, 1/2 cup vegetables, 1/2 cup tuna**
Preparation time: 15 minutes
Cooking time: 10–12 minutes for pasta

SALAD BAR: cherry tomatoes, zucchini, carrots, peppers, red onion, tuna (if available)

ALSO VISIT: shelves for tuna (if not on the salad bar), balsamic vinegar, bottled lemon juice, pasta

1	cup halved cherry tomatoes
1	cup sliced zucchini
1	cup shredded or sliced carrots
1/2	cup red or green bell pepper strips
1/4	cup sliced red onion
2	cups flaked tuna (canned or from salad bar)
1/4	cup balsamic vinegar
2	Tbsp minced fresh basil
2	Tbsp olive oil
1	Tbsp lemon juice
	Fresh ground pepper and salt to taste
4	cups cooked small pasta shells

Combine all ingredients in a large bowl. Chill in the refrigerator for 1 hour.

Exchanges
3 Starch
1 Vegetable
2 Lean Meat

Calories 385
   Calories from Fat . . 77
Total Fat . . . . 9 g
   Saturated Fat . . . . . . 2 g
Cholesterol . . . . 22 mg
Sodium . . . . 280 mg
Carbohydrate . . . . . . 48 g
   Dietary Fiber . . . . . . 4 g
   Sugars . . . . 6 g
Protein . . . . 28 g

Summer Ratatouille

Serves 4   Serving size: 1 cup
Preparation time: 10 minutes
Cooking time: 5 minutes
Standing time: 1 hour

SALAD BAR: zucchini, yellow squash, onion, cherry tomatoes

ALSO VISIT: shelves for eggplant caponata, bottled lemon juice, spices; produce for mint

1	Tbsp olive oil, divided
3	cups combination sliced zucchini and yellow squash
1	cup sliced onion
1	cup halved cherry tomatoes
1/3	cup minced fresh mint leaves
1	Tbsp fresh lemon juice
1	4.75-oz can prepared eggplant caponata
1/4	tsp salt
1/4	tsp fresh ground black pepper

1. In a large skillet over medium-high heat, heat 1/2 Tbsp olive oil. Add the zucchini and yellow squash and onion and sauté for 5–7 minutes until tender, stirring often.

2. Remove the zucchini–yellow squash sauté to a salad bowl. Add remaining ingredients and let stand at room temperature for 1 hour.

Exchanges
2 Vegetable
1 Monounsaturated Fat

Calories 105
 Calories from Fat . . 54
Total Fat . . . . 6 g
 Saturated Fat . . . . . . 1 g
Cholesterol . . . . 0 mg
Sodium . . . . 299 mg
Carbohydrate . . . . . . 11 g
 Dietary Fiber . . . . . . 4 g
 Sugars . . . . 7 g
Protein . . . . 2 g

One-Pot Chicken and Vegetables

Serves 4   Serving size: 4 oz chicken, 1/2 cup vegetables, 1/2 cup rice

Preparation time: 10 minutes

Cooking time: 15 minutes (add 45 minutes if rice is not cooked before preparing the recipe)

SALAD BAR: zucchini, carrot, red onion, celery

ALSO VISIT: shelves for canned tomatoes, rice, spices; meat department for uncooked chicken or deli for precooked chicken

1	Tbsp olive oil
1	cup sliced zucchini
1	cup sliced or shredded carrot
1/2	cup sliced green onions or red onion
1/2	cup sliced celery
1	14 1/2-oz can diced tomatoes
1	lb cooked, diced chicken breasts
1	tsp dried oregano
1/2	tsp dried basil
1/4	tsp salt
1/8	tsp fresh ground black pepper
2	cups cooked brown rice, hot

1. In a skillet over medium-high heat, heat the oil. Add the zucchini, carrots, green or red onion, and celery and sauté for 5 minutes, stirring occasionally.

2. Add the canned diced tomatoes and lower the heat. Simmer for 5 minutes.

3. Add the chicken and seasonings and simmer for 3 minutes.

4. Serve the chicken and vegetables over cooked rice.

Exchanges

2 Starch
1 Vegetable
4 Lean Meat

Calories 406
  Calories from Fat . 121
Total Fat . . . . 13 g
  Saturated Fat . . . . . . 3 g
Cholesterol . . . . 96 mg
Sodium . . . . 409 mg
Carbohydrate . . . . . . 32 g
  Dietary Fiber . . . . . . 5 g
  Sugars . . . . 6 g
Protein . . . . 38 g

Mediterranean Vegetables and Shrimp with Orzo

Serves 4   Serving size: 1/2 cup vegetables, 4 oz shrimp, 1/2 cup orzo

Preparation time: 15 minutes

Cooking time: 10 minutes (add 6–8 minutes for cooking orzo if not prepared before recipe)

SALAD BAR: celery, carrot, zucchini, cherry tomatoes, chickpeas

ALSO VISIT: seafood department or shelves for salad shrimp (either fresh or canned); dairy for feta cheese; shelves for orzo

1	Tbsp olive oil
1/2	cup sliced celery
1	cup broccoli florets
1	cup sliced or shredded carrot
1	cup sliced zucchini
1	cup halved cherry tomatoes
1	tsp dried basil
2	tsp dried oregano
1	cup chickpeas, rinsed and drained
1	lb cooked salad shrimp
2	cups hot cooked orzo pasta
2	oz crumbled feta cheese

1. In a skillet over medium-high heat, heat the oil. Add the celery, broccoli, carrots, and zucchini and sauté for 5 minutes. Add the cherry tomatoes, basil, and oregano. Lower the heat, cover, and cook for 3 minutes until the tomatoes begin to soften. Add the chickpeas and sauté for 1 minute.

2. Add the cooked shrimp and cook for 30 seconds.

3. Serve the vegetable and shrimp mixture over the pasta and top with feta cheese.

Exchanges

3 Starch
1 Vegetable
3 Lean Meat

Calories 440
   Calories from Fat . . 87
Total Fat . . . . 10 g
   Saturated Fat . . . . . . 3 g
Cholesterol . . . . 233 mg
Sodium . . . . 504 mg
Carbohydrate . . . . . . 52 g
   Dietary Fiber . . . . . . 7 g
   Sugars . . . . 9 g
Protein . . . . 36 g

Asian Pasta Stir-Fry

Serves 4   Serving size: 1/2 cup vegetables, 1 cup pasta
Preparation time: 15 minutes
Cooking time: 10 minutes (add 5 minutes if angel hair pasta is not cooked before starting recipe)

SALAD BAR: celery, mushrooms, carrots, broccoli, cauliflower

ALSO VISIT: shelves for hoisin sauce, soy sauce, sherry, angel hair pasta, spices

2	tsp peanut oil
1/2	cup sliced celery
1/2	cup sliced mushrooms
1	cup sliced carrots
2	cups broccoli florets
1	cup cauliflower florets

Sauce:

3	Tbsp bottled hoisin sauce
2	tsp lite soy sauce
2	Tbsp dry sherry
1	tsp sugar
4	cups cooked angel hair pasta

1. In a skillet over medium-high heat, heat the oil. Add the celery and mushrooms and sauté for 5 minutes. Add the carrots, broccoli, and cauliflower. Cover and lower heat to simmer for 4 minutes, adding water if necessary to keep the vegetables moist.

2. Combine all the sauce ingredients in a small bowl. Add to the vegetables and cook for 1 minute.

3. Serve the vegetables and sauce over the pasta.

Exchanges
3 1/2 Starch
1 Vegetable

Calories 283
    Calories from Fat . . 32
Total Fat . . . . 4 g
    Saturated Fat . . . . . . 1 g
Cholesterol . . . . 0 mg
Sodium . . . . 377 mg
Carbohydrate . . . . . . 56 g
    Dietary Fiber . . . . . . 6 g
    Sugars . . . . 10 g
Protein . . . . 9 g

Stir-Fry Vegetable Wraps

Serves 4   Serving size: 1 wrap (1 tortilla, 3/4 cup vegetables)
Preparation time: 15 minutes
Cooking time: 5 minutes

SALAD BAR: green onion, carrots, zucchini or yellow squash, cabbage, mushrooms, bean sprouts

ALSO VISIT: produce section for ginger; refrigerated section for tortillas; shelves for sesame oil, hoisin sauce, soy sauce

2 tsp sesame oil

2 tsp minced ginger root

2 Tbsp minced green onion

1 cup shredded carrots

1 cup finely diced zucchini or yellow squash

1 cup shredded cabbage

1 cup chopped mushrooms

1 cup bean sprouts

4 10-inch whole-wheat tortillas

4 tsp hoisin sauce

2 tsp lite soy sauce

1. In a wok or large skillet over high heat, heat the oil. Add the ginger and green onion and stir-fry for 30 seconds.

2. Add the carrots, zucchini or yellow squash, cabbage, and mushrooms and stir-fry for 2–3 minutes.

3. Add the bean sprouts and stir-fry for 1 minute.

4. Combine the hoisin sauce and soy sauce. Spread some of this mixture over each tortilla. Divide the vegetables among the tortillas. Fold over sides of each tortilla and roll up.

Exchanges
2 Starch
2 Vegetable
1 Fat

Calories 253
    Calories from Fat . . 66
Total Fat . . . . 7 g
    Saturated Fat . . . . . . 2 g
Cholesterol . . . . 0 mg
Sodium . . . . 636 mg
Carbohydrate . . . . . . 40 g
    Dietary Fiber . . . . . . 4 g
    Sugars . . . . 6 g
Protein . . . . 7 g

Bow Tie Noodles with Marinated Vegetable Sauce

Serves 4   Serving size: 1 cup pasta, 1 1/4 cup sauce
Preparation time: 15 minutes
Cooking time: 10–12 minutes
Standing time: 1 hour

SALAD BAR: peppers, zucchini, celery, onion, cherry tomatoes, carrots

ALSO VISIT: produce for basil, parsley, oregano; shelves for balsamic vinegar, lemon juice, bow tie noodles, spices; refrigerated section for cheese

1 cup diced red or green bell peppers

1 cup sliced zucchini

1/2 cup sliced celery

1/2 cup sliced onions

1 cup halved cherry tomatoes

1 cup sliced or shredded carrots

2 Tbsp olive oil

3 Tbsp balsamic vinegar

2 Tbsp lemon juice

2 Tbsp minced fresh basil

2 Tbsp minced fresh parsley

2 tsp minced fresh oregano

1/4 tsp salt

1/4 tsp fresh ground black pepper

1/4 cup fresh grated Parmesan cheese

4 cups cooked bow tie noodles

Exchanges

3 Starch
1 Vegetable
1 1/2 Monounsaturated Fat

Calories 335
  Calories from Fat . . 93
Total Fat . . . . 10 g
  Saturated Fat . . . . . . 3 g
Cholesterol . . . . 8 mg
Sodium . . . . 307 mg
Carbohydrate . . . . . . 51 g
  Dietary Fiber . . . . . . 5 g
  Sugars . . . . 7 g
Protein . . . . 11 g

1. In a large bowl, mix together peppers, zucchini, celery, onions, cherry tomatoes, and carrots. Add oil, vinegar, and lemon juice. Place mixture in refrigerator and chill for 1 hour.

2. Remove mixture from refrigerator and add herbs, pepper, and salt. Mix cheese and pasta together. Top each serving with some vegetable sauce.

Rigatoni and Roasted Vegetables

Serves 4   Serving size: 1 cup pasta, 1/4 of recipe vegetables
Preparation time: 15 minutes
Cooking time: 10 minutes (add 10–12 minutes for rigatoni if not
cooked before starting recipe)

SALAD BAR: peppers, mushrooms, zucchini, cherry tomatoes

ALSO VISIT: shelves for rigatoni, Italian salad dressing

- 2   cups red or green bell pepper strips
- 1   cup sliced mushrooms
- 1   cup sliced zucchini
- 1   cup halved cherry tomatoes
- 2   Tbsp olive oil or flavored olive oil
- 4   cups cooked rigatoni
- 1/2   cup fat-free Italian salad dressing

1. Preheat the oven broiler. Line a rack with foil and place 5 inches from the heat source. Brush the vegetables with olive oil and place on the rack.

2. Broil the vegetables for about 10 minutes until slightly charred. Remove them from the oven.

3. Toss the vegetables with cooked pasta. Add the salad dressing and toss well. Serve warm or chill and serve cold.

Exchanges

3 Starch
1 Vegetable
1 Monounsaturated Fat

Calories 303
  Calories from Fat . . 73
Total Fat . . . . 8 g
  Saturated Fat . . . . . . 2 g
Cholesterol . . . . 0 mg
Sodium . . . . 319 mg
Carbohydrate . . . . . . 49 g
  Dietary Fiber . . . . . . 4 g
  Sugars . . . . 7 g
Protein . . . . 8 g

Marinated Chickpea and Tuna Salad

Serves 4   Serving size: 1/2 cup tuna, 1 cup vegetables, 1/2 cup chickpeas

Preparation time: 15 minutes

Standing time: 1 hour

SALAD BAR: chickpeas, peppers, cherry tomatoes, celery, green onions, carrots, tuna (if available)

ALSO VISIT: shelves for vinegar, tuna (if not on salad bar), spices; produce for rosemary, basil

2	cups chickpeas, rinsed and drained
2	cups red or green bell pepper strips
1	cup halved cherry tomatoes
1/2	cup sliced celery
2	Tbsp sliced green onions
1	cup sliced or shredded carrots
2	cups tuna (canned or from the salad bar)
2	Tbsp regular or garlic-flavored olive oil
1/4	cup balsamic or red wine vinegar
1	tsp minced fresh rosemary
2	Tbsp minced fresh basil
1/8	tsp salt
1/8	tsp fresh ground black pepper

Combine all ingredients in a salad bowl. Refrigerate for 1 hour before serving.

Exchanges

1 1/2 Starch
2 Vegetable
3 Very Lean Meat
1 Monounsaturated Fat

Calories	325
Calories from Fat	88
Total Fat	10 g
Saturated Fat	2 g
Cholesterol	22 mg
Sodium	483 mg
Carbohydrate	32 g
Dietary Fiber	9 g
Sugars	7 g
Protein	28 g

Chinese Stir-Fried Cherry Tomatoes and Carrots with Shrimp

Serves 4   **Serving size: 3 oz shrimp, 1/2 cup vegetables, 1/2 cup rice**
Preparation time: 15 minutes   **Cooking time: 7–8 minutes**

SALAD BAR: green onions, cherry tomatoes, carrots

ALSO VISIT: produce for ginger, garlic; shelves for soy sauce, vinegar, rice; frozen foods for shrimp

2	tsp canola oil
1	tsp sesame oil
1	tsp minced ginger
1	tsp minced garlic
2	Tbsp sliced green onions
3	cups halved cherry tomatoes
1 1/2	cups sliced or shredded carrots
1	Tbsp lite soy sauce
2	tsp rice vinegar
1	lb cooked medium shrimp, peeled and deveined
2	cups cooked brown rice, hot

1. In a wok over high heat, heat the two oils. Reduce heat to medium-high. Add ginger, garlic, and green onions and stir-fry 30 seconds. Add cherry tomatoes and stir-fry 2 minutes. Add carrots and stir-fry 2 minutes.

2. Add soy sauce and rice vinegar and stir-fry 1 minute. Add shrimp and stir-fry 1 minute. Serve tomato-shrimp mixture over brown rice.

Exchanges

1 1/2 Starch
2 Vegetable
3 Very Lean Meat
1/2 Monounsaturated Fat

Calories 305
  Calories from Fat . . 55
Total Fat . . . . 6 g
  Saturated Fat . . . . . . 0 g
Cholesterol . . . . 220 mg
Sodium . . . . 437 mg
Carbohydrate . . . . . . 35 g
  Dietary Fiber . . . . . . 5 g
  Sugars . . . . 8 g
Protein . . . . 28 g

Italian Tuna Pizzas

Serves 4 Serving size: 1 pita, 1/4 cup sauce, 1/4 cup vegetables, 1/4 cup tuna
Preparation time: 15 minutes
Cooking time: 15 minutes

SALAD BAR: peppers, zucchini, green onion, tuna (if available)

ALSO VISIT: dairy for cheese; shelves for tomato sauce, olives, tuna (if not on salad bar), spices; bread department for pita

1	Tbsp olive oil
2	cups red or green bell pepper strips
1/2	cup sliced zucchini
2	Tbsp sliced green onion
4	6-inch whole-wheat pita breads
1	cup favorite tomato sauce
1	cup flaked tuna
1	cup part-skim mozzarella cheese
1/2	cup sliced black olives
1	tsp dried oregano
1	tsp dried basil

1. Preheat the oven to 400°F. In a skillet over medium-high heat, heat the oil. Add the pepper strips, zucchini, and green onion. Sauté for 5 minutes, stirring occasionally. Set aside.

2. Spread the tomato sauce evenly over all four pita breads.

3. Arrange the tuna and vegetables over the tomato sauce. Divide the cheese equally among the pitas. Sprinkle with olives, oregano, and basil.

4. Place the pita pizzas on a baking sheet. Bake for 7–9 minutes until cheese melts and pitas are hot.

Exchanges

2 Starch
2 Vegetable
2 Lean Meat
1/2 Monounsaturated Fat

Calories 346
  Calories from Fat . 108
Total Fat . . . . 12 g
  Saturated Fat . . . . . . 4 g
Cholesterol . . . . 27 mg
Sodium . . . . 790 mg
Carbohydrate . . . . . . 27 g
  Dietary Fiber . . . . . . 5 g
  Sugars . . . . 7 g
Protein . . . . 24 g

Fresh Tomato and Cucumber Salsa with Roasted Turkey

Serves 4   Serving size: 4 oz turkey, 2/3 cup salsa
Preparation time: 10 minutes
Standing time: 1 hour

SALAD BAR: cherry tomatoes, cucumbers, green onion

ALSO VISIT: produce for garlic, cilantro; shelves for vinegar, spices; deli or meat department for turkey

2	cups halved cherry tomatoes
1	cup diced cucumber
2	Tbsp sliced green onion
1	tsp minced garlic
1/2	tsp sugar
2	tsp red wine vinegar
1	tsp dry oregano
1	tsp minced fresh cilantro
1/4	tsp salt
1/4	tsp fresh ground black pepper
1	lb sliced roasted turkey breast

1. Combine all the salsa ingredients and place in the refrigerator to chill for 1 hour.

2. Serve the salsa with slices of hot or cold roasted turkey breast.

Exchanges
1 Vegetable
4 Very Lean Meat

Calories 179
    Calories from Fat . . 10
Total Fat . . . . 1 g
    Saturated Fat . . . . . . 0 g
Cholesterol . . . . 92 mg
Sodium . . . . 215 mg
Carbohydrate . . . . 6 g
    Dietary Fiber . . . . . . 1 g
    Sugars . . . . 4 g
Protein . . . . 35 g

Cool Melon and Shrimp Salad

Serves 4   Serving size: 4 oz shrimp, 1/4 cup fruit
Preparation time: 15 minutes
Chilling time: several hours (optional)

SALAD BAR: melon, cucumber, green onions

ALSO VISIT: frozen foods for shrimp, limeade concentrate; shelves for spices

- 1/2 cup honeydew chunks
- 1/2 cup cantaloupe chunks
- 1 cup sliced cucumber (in bite-sized pieces)
- 1/4 cup sliced green onions
- 1 lb frozen, precooked large shrimp, thawed

Dressing:
- 1/2 cup limeade concentrate
- 2 tsp canola oil
- 1 tsp chili powder

1. Combine the melons, cucumbers, green onions, and shrimp.

2. In a small bowl, whisk together the dressing ingredients. Add to the fruit–shrimp mixture.

3. Serve at room temperature or chill for several hours.

Exchanges
1 1/2 Carbohydrate
4 Very Lean Meat

Calories 222
  Calories from Fat . . 34
Total Fat . . . . 4 g
  Saturated Fat . . . . . . 0 g
Cholesterol . . . . 220 mg
Sodium . . . . 264 mg
Carbohydrate . . . . . . 23 g
  Dietary Fiber . . . . . . 1 g
  Sugars . . . . 20 g
Protein . . . . 24 g

Leftover Stir-Fry

Serves 6   Serving size: 3–4 oz meat, 1/2 cup vegetables, 1/2 cup rice

Preparation time: 20 minutes

SALAD BAR: assorted sliced vegetables

ALSO VISIT: meat department for chicken; shelves for soy sauce, brown sugar, sherry, rice, sesame seeds

> 1 Tbsp peanut oil
>
> 1 1/2 lb boneless, skinless chicken breasts or lean sirloin steak (either raw or cooked, see directions), sliced into strips
>
> 3 cups sliced vegetables (carrots, broccoli, zucchini, peppers)
>
> 2 garlic cloves, minced
>
> 2 Tbsp lite soy sauce
>
> 2 Tbsp brown sugar
>
> 1 Tbsp dry sherry
>
> 3 cups cooked rice

Garnish: 2 Tbsp toasted sesame seeds

1. In a wok over high heat, heat the oil. If using raw meat, add the chicken breasts or sirloin, reduce the heat to medium-high, and stir-fry the chicken for 5 minutes or the steak for 4–5 minutes. If using precooked chicken or steak, start with step 2, using the oil to stir-fry the vegetables.

2. Add the vegetables and stir-fry for 4 minutes. Add the garlic and stir-fry for 2 more minutes. Add the chicken or beef at this point if using precooked meat.

3. Combine the soy sauce, sugar, and sherry. Add to the wok. Cover and steam for 1 minute. Serve over cooked rice, and garnish with sesame seeds.

Exchanges (calculated using precooked meat)

2 Starch
4 Lean Meat

Calories	381
Calories from Fat	88
Total Fat	10 g
Saturated Fat	3 g
Cholesterol	98 mg
Sodium	293 mg
Carbohydrate	32 g
Dietary Fiber	2 g
Sugars	7 g
Protein	38 g

Creamy Vegetable Soup

Serves 4   Serving size: 1 cup
Preparation time: 30 minutes

SALAD BAR: cauliflower, broccoli, celery, onion

ALSO VISIT: shelves for broth, mustard, evaporated skimmed milk, cornstarch; produce for dill, parsley

1	Tbsp olive oil
3	garlic cloves, minced
1	cup chopped cauliflower
1	cup chopped broccoli
1/2	cup chopped carrot
1/4	cup chopped celery
1/2	cup chopped onion
1	14.5-oz can low-fat, low-sodium chicken broth
2	Tbsp Dijon mustard
1	12-oz can evaporated skimmed milk
	Fresh ground pepper and salt to taste
1	Tbsp minced fresh dill
2	tsp minced fresh parsley
1	Tbsp cornstarch or arrowroot powder
2	Tbsp water

Garnish: 1/4 cup Parmesan cheese

1. In a stockpot over medium heat, heat the oil. Add the garlic and sauté for 30 seconds. Add the cauliflower, broccoli, carrot, celery, and onion and sauté for 10 minutes.

2. Add half of the can of broth to the stockpot and bring to a boil. Simmer for 10 minutes.

3. In batches, puree the cooked vegetables in the blender. Set aside in a separate bowl.

Exchanges
1 1/2 Carbohydrate
1/2 Monounsaturated Fat

Calories 157
  Calories from Fat . . 37
Total Fat . . . . 4 g
  Saturated Fat . . . . . . 1 g
Cholesterol . . . . 3 mg
Sodium . . . . 496 mg
Carbohydrate . . . . . . 20 g
  Dietary Fiber . . . . . . 2 g
  Sugars . . . . 13 g
Protein . . . . 11 g

4. In the same stockpot, heat the remaining broth with the mustard, evaporated milk, and salt and pepper. Bring to a gentle simmer. Add the pureed vegetables and simmer on low for 5 minutes. Add the herbs and simmer for 2 minutes. Mix together the cornstarch or arrowroot with the water. Add to the soup and cook for 2 minutes until thickened.

5. Divide into bowls and garnish with cheese to serve.

Salad Bar Chicken Salad with Peanut Sauce

Serves 4   Serving size: 4 oz chicken, 1 cup vegetables
Preparation time: 20 minutes

SALAD BAR: celery, mushrooms, carrots, red bell pepper, bean sprouts, green onions

ALSO VISIT: deli for cooked chicken breast; shelves for broth, peanut butter, soy sauce, spices, arrowroot, sesame seeds

- 1 lb cooked chicken, cut into 2-inch strips
- 1 cup diagonally sliced celery
- 1/2 cup thinly sliced mushrooms
- 1 cup thinly sliced carrots, sliced diagonally
- 1/2 cup thinly sliced red bell pepper
- 1 cup bean sprouts
- 1 cup low-sodium, low-fat chicken broth
- 2 Tbsp peanut butter
- 4 Tbsp lite soy sauce
- 1 tsp garlic powder
- 1 tsp crushed red pepper
- 1 tsp ground ginger
- 1 Tbsp arrowroot or cornstarch
- 2 Tbsp water

Garnish: 2 Tbsp toasted sesame seeds; 1/2 cup minced green onions

1. Combine first 6 ingredients in a large bowl. In a medium saucepan over medium heat, combine all remaining ingredients except for arrowroot and water. Bring to a boil, then reduce the heat and simmer for 5 minutes.

2. Combine arrowroot and water. Add to sauce mixture. Bring to a boil and simmer until thickened, about 3 minutes. Pour sauce over salad. Garnish with sesame seeds and green onions and serve.

Exchanges
1 Carbohydrate
4 Lean Meat

Calories 286
  Calories from Fat . . 75
Total Fat . . . . 8 g
  Saturated Fat . . . . . . 2 g
Cholesterol . . . . 96 mg
Sodium . . . . 921 mg
Carbohydrate . . . . . . 12 g
  Dietary Fiber . . . . . . 3 g
  Sugars . . . . 6 g
Protein . . . . 40 g

Recipes from the Deli

IF YOU ARE FROM NEW YORK LIKE I AM, you practically grew up on deli food. Back then, we weren't as aware of the link between high fat and sodium intake and heart disease. Today, instead of fatty corned beef and pastrami, many delis stock low-fat sliced meats and fresh roasted chickens and game hens. With careful selection, you can put many of your supermarket's deli items to good use!

Look for delis that offer real sliced meats, not the pressed versions of them. Always pull the skin off the rotisserie chickens or purchase them skinless if you can. Even marinated vegetable salads can be part of recipes—just drain off most of the oil. The deli is often a great place to purchase specialty foods like roasted peppers, olives, and artichoke hearts when you just don't need to buy a whole can.

Like salad bars, make sure you visit a deli that you know sells fresh items. Use deli meat up in no more than 3 days for best freshness. Once you unwrap deli meat, be sure to rewrap it tightly in butcher or waxed paper and place it in a zippered plastic bag before refrigerating.

Make sure you ask about the nutritional facts when purchasing deli meats. Some lean products will be identified as fat-free, low-fat, or lean. Remember a good rule of thumb in choosing low-fat products: for every 100 calories, the product should not have more than 2–3 grams of fat.

Be aware that deli meats often are high in sodium, so ask for low-sodium varieties if available. Smoked meats will definitely be higher in sodium than unsmoked products. If you are watching your sodium intake, you may prefer to roast your own meat and freeze it in individual serving packets for easy meal preparation.

*R*ecipes

Apricot-Orange Chicken with Glazed Onions

Serves 4   Serving size: 1/4 chicken
Preparation time: 10 minutes
Cooking time: 35 minutes

DELI: chicken

ALSO VISIT: shelves for preserves, marmalade, vinegar; produce for onion, garlic

1 whole roasted deli chicken, skinned
3 Tbsp no-added-sugar apricot preserves, divided
3 Tbsp no-added-sugar orange marmalade, divided
2 Tbsp balsamic vinegar, divided
   Nonstick cooking spray
1 large onion, quartered
1 clove garlic, minced

1. Preheat oven to 375°F. In small bowl, blend 1 Tbsp each apricot preserves, marmalade, and vinegar.

2. Place chicken in baking pan coated with nonstick cooking spray. Add water to pan to a depth of 1/4–1/2 inch. Brush chicken with preserve mixture. Combine the remaining preserves, marmalade, vinegar, onion, and garlic and spoon around the chicken.

3. Roast, covered, for 25 minutes. Uncover and roast for 10 more minutes, until onion is tender.

Exchanges
1 Carbohydrate
4 Lean Meat

Calories 278
  Calories from Fat . . 77
Total Fat . . . . 9 g
  Saturated Fat . . . . . . 2 g
Cholesterol . . . . 100 mg
Sodium . . . . 110 mg
Carbohydrate . . . . . . 15 g
  Dietary Fiber . . . . . . 1 g
  Sugars . . . . 10 g
Protein . . . . 34 g

Roasted Potatoes, Chicken, and Cheese

Serves 4   Serving size: 1 3/4 cups
Preparation time: 15 minutes
Cooking time: about 1 hour

DELI: smoked chicken

ALSO VISIT: produce for potatoes, garlic; shelves for spices, vinegar; dairy case for cheese

Nonstick cooking spray
4 large red potatoes, scrubbed and quartered
Black pepper to taste
2 tsp minced garlic
2 Tbsp olive oil
1 Tbsp Italian seasonings
1/4 cup fat-free Parmesan cheese, shredded
2 cups smoked deli chicken, diced (or use regular cooked chicken to reduce sodium)
1/4 cup balsamic vinegar
1/4 cup water

1. Preheat oven to 350°F. Spray a glass baking dish with nonstick spray.

2. Combine ingredients in a large bowl. Pour into the glass baking dish and cover with foil. Bake for 45 minutes. Uncover and bake for 10–15 minutes more, until potatoes are tender.

Exchanges
2 Starch
2 Lean Meat

Calories 267
    Calories from Fat . . 68
Total Fat . . . . 8 g
    Saturated Fat . . . . . . 2 g
Cholesterol . . . . 33 mg
Sodium . . . . 965 mg
Carbohydrate . . . . . . 29 g
    Dietary Fiber . . . . . . 3 g
    Sugars . . . . 6 g
Protein . . . . 20 g

Toasted Vegetable Baguette

Serves 4 Serving size: 1 baguette, 1/4 lb salad, 1 slice cheese (approx. 2 oz)
Preparation time: 5 minutes
Cooking time: 2 minutes

DELI: vegetable salad

ALSO VISIT: bread department for baguettes; dairy for cheese; produce for parsley

4	6-inch mini-baguettes cut lengthwise
1	lb roasted vegetable salad, drained
1/4	cup chopped parsley
4	2-oz slices provolone cheese

1. Preheat oven to 350°F.

2. Open each baguette and fill with vegetable salad. Sprinkle on 1/4 of parsley, and lay a slice of provolone cheese over the top. Close sandwich.

3. Place sandwiches on a baking sheet and bake for 5 minutes, until cheese melts.

Exchanges
2 Starch
1 Vegetable
2 Medium-Fat Meat
1 Saturated Fat

Calories	388
Calories from Fat	. 153
Total Fat	17 g
Saturated Fat	10 g
Cholesterol	40 mg
Sodium	884 mg
Carbohydrate	38 g
Dietary Fiber	2 g
Sugars	3 g
Protein	21 g

Asparagus, Smoked Turkey, and Cashew Stir-Fry

Serves 4 Serving size: 1 1/4 cups
Preparation time: 10 minutes
Cooking time: 7–8 minutes

DELI: smoked turkey

ALSO VISIT: frozen foods for asparagus; produce for garlic, lemon; shelves for spices

1	10-oz pkg frozen asparagus, thawed
1	Tbsp canola oil
1	tsp minced garlic
1	Tbsp freshly squeezed lemon juice
1/2	tsp dried marjoram
2	Tbsp toasted chopped cashew nuts
1	lb smoked deli turkey, sliced about 1/2 inch thick (or use regular cooked turkey to reduce sodium)
	Salt and fresh ground pepper to taste

1. Slice asparagus diagonally and set aside.
2. In a wok or large skillet over medium heat, heat the oil.
3. Add garlic, lemon juice, dried marjoram, cashews, smoked turkey, and salt and pepper to taste. Stir-fry for 5 minutes until heated through.
4. Add the asparagus and stir-fry for 2–3 minutes more. Asparagus should retain its color.

Exchanges
1 Vegetable
3 Very Lean Meat
1 Monounsaturated Fat

Calories 179
    Calories from Fat . . 64
Total Fat . . . . 7 g
    Saturated Fat . . . . . . 1 g
Cholesterol . . . . 52 mg
Sodium . . . . 1393 mg
Carbohydrate . . . . 5 g
    Dietary Fiber . . . . . . 1 g
    Sugars . . . . 2 g
Protein . . . . 25 g

Pea, Tomato, and Ham Salad

Serves 4   Serving size: 1 1/3 cups
Preparation time: 10 minutes
Standing time: 1 hour

DELI: ham

ALSO VISIT: frozen foods for peas; shelves for vinegar, spices

- 1 1-lb pkg frozen peas, thawed (put in colander and run hot water over the peas to thaw)
- 1 14.5-oz can diced tomatoes, well drained
- 1/2 tsp cumin

  Salt and fresh ground pepper to taste

- 1 Tbsp mustard vinegar (if not available, use 1/2 Tbsp Dijon mustard and 1/2 Tbsp white wine vinegar)
- 1 cup diced baked ham

1. Combine all ingredients in a large bowl. Mix gently but thoroughly. Chill for at least 1 hour before serving.

Exchanges

1 Starch
2 Very Lean Meat

Calories 166
   Calories from Fat . . 33
Total Fat . . . . 4 g
   Saturated Fat . . . . . . 1 g
Cholesterol . . . . 32 mg
Sodium . . . . 306 mg
Carbohydrate . . . . . . 18 g
   Dietary Fiber . . . . . . 6 g
   Sugars . . . . 8 g
Protein . . . . 16 g

Mexican Dinner Rice

Serves 4   Serving size: 1 cup
Preparation time: 15 minutes   Cooking time: 45 minutes

DELI: turkey

ALSO VISIT: shelves for broth, rice, stewed tomatoes, chilies, spices, hot sauce; salad bar or produce section for onion, bell peppers; frozen foods for corn; produce for garlic

- 1 Tbsp olive oil
- 1 Tbsp + 1/2 cup low-fat, low-sodium chicken broth
- 1/3 cup long-grain brown rice
- 1 Tbsp chopped garlic
- 1/2 cup chopped onion
- 1/4 cup chopped green bell pepper
- 1/4 cup chopped red bell pepper
- 1 can (14.5 oz) chopped stewed tomatoes, in their own juices
- 1 can (4 oz) green chilies, chopped, not drained
- 3/4 cup frozen kernel corn
- 1/2 pkg taco seasoning (or 1 tsp chili powder to reduce sodium)
- 1 tsp green hot sauce (add more or less depending on how spicy you want it)
- 1 1/2 cups chopped cooked deli turkey breast

1. In a large nonstick skillet over medium heat sauté oil, 1 Tbsp chicken broth, rice, garlic, onion, and peppers for 4–5 minutes, until rice is browned and onions are translucent.

2. Stir in tomatoes, remaining 1/2 cup chicken broth, green chilies, corn, taco seasoning, and hot sauce and bring to a boil. Reduce heat to low, cover, and simmer for 35 minutes.

3. Add turkey and cook for 5 more minutes until rice is tender.

Exchanges

1 1/2 Starch
2 Vegetable
2 Very Lean Meat

Calories	244
Calories from Fat	42
Total Fat	5 g
Saturated Fat	1 g
Cholesterol	43 mg
Sodium	695 mg
Carbohydrate	31 g
Dietary Fiber	4 g
Sugars	6 g
Protein	20 g

Mexican Chicken

Serves 4   Serving size: 3–4 oz chicken, 6 oz sauce
Preparation time: 10 minutes
Cooking time: 45 minutes

DELI: salsa

ALSO VISIT: dairy case for sour cream, cheese; meat department for chicken; shelves for spices; produce for cilantro

2	cups deli fresh salsa
1/4	cup chopped cilantro
1	cup fat-free sour cream
1/4	cup low-fat shredded cheddar cheese
1/2	pkg taco seasoning (or 1–2 tsp chili powder to reduce sodium)
	Nonstick cooking spray
4	4-oz boneless, skinless chicken breasts

1. Preheat oven to 350°F.

2. In a mixing bowl, mix together salsa, cilantro, sour cream, cheddar cheese, and taco seasoning.

3. Place chicken into a glass baking dish sprayed with nonstick cooking spray. Pour sauce over chicken and bake 40–45 minutes, until the chicken registers 170°F on an instant thermometer.

Exchanges
1 1/2 Carbohydrate
4 Very Lean Meat

Calories 250
  Calories from Fat . . 31
Total Fat . . . . 3 g
  Saturated Fat . . . . . . 1 g
Cholesterol . . . . 74 mg
Sodium . . . . 1281 mg
Carbohydrate . . . . . . 24 g
  Dietary Fiber . . . . . . 1 g
  Sugars . . . . 13 g
Protein . . . . 30 g

Stuffed Tomatoes with Smoked Chicken and Tabouli

Serves 4   Serving size: 1 tomato, 6 oz tabouli mixture
Preparation time: 15 minutes
Standing time: 2 hours

DELI: tabouli, hummus, chicken

ALSO VISIT: salad bar or produce for cucumbers; produce for whole tomatoes

- 1 cup deli tabouli
- 1 cup diced, seeded cucumber
- 1 cup diced smoked chicken breast
- 4 medium ripe, firm tomatoes
- 2 tsp olive oil
- 4 Tbsp deli hummus

1. Add the cucumber and chicken to the prepared tabouli mixture and refrigerate for at least 1 hour.

2. Take each tomato and cut off the top (set aside). Scoop out the pulp and discard. Fill the cavity with the tabouli mixture. Drizzle 1/2 tsp olive oil over each tomato and put 1 Tbsp hummus on top of that. Cover the filled tomato with the tomato top and refrigerate for at least 1 hour before serving.

Exchanges

1 Starch
1 Vegetable
1 Very Lean Meat
1/2 Monounsaturated Fat

Calories 158
    Calories from Fat . . 49
Total Fat . . . . 5 g
    Saturated Fat . . . . . . 1 g
Cholesterol . . . . 16 mg
Sodium . . . . 572 mg
Carbohydrate . . . . . . 18 g
    Dietary Fiber . . . . . . 4 g
    Sugars . . . . 6 g
Protein . . . . 10 g

Salmon with Roasted Vegetable Salad

Serves 4   Serving size: 2–3 oz salmon, 1/2 cup salad
Preparation time: 5 minutes
Cooking time: 7–9 minutes

DELI: roasted vegetable salad

ALSO VISIT: shelves for sugar, mustard; seafood department for salmon

> 2 6-oz salmon steaks, deboned
>
> 2 tsp canola oil
>
> 3 Tbsp brown sugar
>
> 1/4 cup Dijon mustard
>
> 2 cups deli roasted vegetable salad (preferably in balsamic vinegar; if in oil, drain oil off)

1. Sprinkle salmon with vegetable oil.

2. In a small bowl, mix together brown sugar and mustard.

3. Set the oven to broil or prepare a grill on a medium-high setting. Broil or grill salmon for 5 minutes. Drizzle the brown sugar and mustard mixture over the salmon. Continue to broil/grill for 2 more minutes. Let the salmon cool for 15 minutes and then cut into bite-sized chunks.

4. In a large bowl, gently mix salmon with roasted vegetable salad. Refrigerate for 30 minutes before serving. Serve on a bed of salad greens, rice, or pasta.

Exchanges
1 Carbohydrate
2 Medium-Fat Meat
1/2 Monounsaturated Fat

Calories 250
    Calories from Fat . 107
Total Fat . . . . 12 g
    Saturated Fat . . . . . . 3 g
Cholesterol . . . . 58 mg
Sodium . . . . 247 mg
Carbohydrate . . . . . . 16 g
    Dietary Fiber . . . . . . 1 g
    Sugars . . . . 12 g
Protein . . . . 19 g

Smoked Chicken with Parmesan Spinach Couscous

Serves 4   Serving size: 1 1/4 cups
Preparation time: 15 minutes
Cooking time: 6 minutes

DELI: chicken

ALSO VISIT: shelves for broth, pine nuts, couscous; produce for basil, garlic; salad bar or produce for spinach; dairy case for cheese

1	tsp olive oil
1	can (14.5 oz) low-fat, low-sodium chicken broth, divided
2	cups cubed smoked chicken
2	tsp chopped garlic
1/4	cup pine nuts
2	cups lightly packed, cleaned, chopped fresh spinach leaves
1	box (5.9 oz) Parmesan couscous
1/4	cup fat-free grated Parmesan cheese
1/4	cup cleaned, chopped fresh basil

1. In a saucepan over medium-high heat, heat the olive oil and 2 Tbsp of chicken broth.

2. Add the diced chicken and garlic. Sauté for about 3 minutes, stirring occasionally.

3. Add pine nuts and continue to brown. When the chicken is browned, add remaining chicken broth, spinach leaves, and spice sack from couscous. Bring to a boil, then reduce heat and add Parmesan cheese and couscous.

4. Remove from heat and let stand 5 minutes. Add basil and lightly fluff couscous with a fork before serving.

Exchanges
2 1/2 Starch
3 Very Lean Meat
1/2 Fat

Calories 334
    Calories from Fat . . 83
Total Fat . . . . 9 g
    Saturated Fat . . . . . . 3 g
Cholesterol . . . . 40 mg
Sodium . . . . 1576 mg
Carbohydrate . . . . . . 37 g
    Dietary Fiber . . . . . . 4 g
    Sugars . . . . 5 g
Protein . . . . 27 g

Deli Chicken Gyro

Serves 4   **Serving size: 1 sandwich (1 pita, 3 oz chicken, 1/2 oz greens and cheese, 2 Tbsp sauce)**

Preparation time: 10 minutes

Standing time: 2 hours

DELI: chicken

ALSO VISIT: salad bar or produce for tomatoes, lettuce, green onion, cucumber, onion; produce for garlic; dairy case for yogurt, feta cheese; bread department for pita bread

        4 pieces whole-wheat pita bread (6-inch diameter)

Sauce:
        1 cup fat-free yogurt with excess water drained

        1 tsp minced garlic

    1/2 cup seeded, diced cucumber

        1 Tbsp finely minced onion

Filling:
      12 oz sliced smoked chicken (or use regular cooked chicken to reduce sodium)

    3/4 cup seeded, diced tomatoes

    1/2 cup shredded lettuce

    1/2 cup feta cheese

    1/2 cup chopped green onion

1. In a mixing bowl, combine yogurt, garlic, cucumber, and onion. Refrigerate 2–3 hours and drain any excess water before serving.

2. Warm pitas in toaster oven or oven. Divide chicken and other gyro filling ingredients onto pitas. Top each pita with 2 Tbsp sauce and fold into a pocket. You may wish to wrap the bottom of each gyro in foil before serving.

Exchanges

2 Starch
1 Vegetable
3 Very Lean Meat

Calories 299
  Calories from Fat . . 49
Total Fat . . . . 5 g
  Saturated Fat . . . . . . 2 g
Cholesterol . . . . 53 mg
Sodium . . . . 1362 mg
Carbohydrate . . . . . . 38 g
  Dietary Fiber . . . . . . 3 g
  Sugars . . . . 9 g
Protein . . . . 28 g

Roasted Turkey, Artichoke, and Couscous Salad

Serves 4   Serving size: 2 cups
Preparation time: 15 minutes
Standing time: 1 hour

DELI: turkey

ALSO VISIT: shelves for artichoke hearts, mushrooms, pine nuts, couscous; salad bar or produce section for tomatoes, green onions; produce for garlic

1	5.9-oz box couscous, prepared as directed but omitting oil and salt
1	lb roasted deli turkey breast, cut into strips (or use regular cooked turkey to reduce sodium)
1	6-oz jar artichoke hearts, drained and halved
1/4	cup chopped green onion
1	tsp minced garlic
1	6-oz jar marinated mushrooms (vinegar marinade), undrained (if in oil, drain off oil)
1	cup chopped tomatoes
1/4	cup toasted pine nuts
1	Tbsp olive oil

1. In a large bowl, combine turkey breast, artichoke hearts, green onions, garlic, marinated mushrooms (marinade included), chopped tomatoes, toasted pine nuts, prepared couscous, and olive oil.

2. Mix thoroughly and refrigerate for at least 1 hour before serving.

Exchanges
2 1/2 Starch
1 Vegetable
3 Lean Meat

Calories 399
  Calories from Fat . 111
Total Fat . . . . 12 g
  Saturated Fat . . . . . . 3 g
Cholesterol . . . . 52 mg
Sodium . . . . 1105 mg
Carbohydrate . . . . . . 42 g
  Dietary Fiber . . . . . . 4 g
  Sugars . . . . 4 g
Protein . . . . 33 g

Smoked Chicken Chili Rellenos

Serves 6   Serving size: 2 chilies with 1 1/3 cups filling and cheeses
Preparation time: 15 minutes
Cooking time: 25 minutes

DELI: chicken

ALSO VISIT: shelves for chilies, flour, salsa; dairy case for milk, cheeses, eggs, egg substitute

	Nonstick cooking spray
4	cans (4 oz each) whole green chilies, seeds removed, slit on one side and opened flat
1	lb smoked chicken cut into 1/2-inch strips (or use regular cooked chicken to reduce sodium)
1	cup reduced-fat Monterey Jack cheese with jalapeños, shredded
1/4	cup egg substitute
2	eggs
1/2	cup flour
	Salt and fresh ground pepper to taste
1/2	cup fat-free milk
1/2	cup salsa
1/2	cup reduced-fat shredded cheddar cheese

1. Preheat oven to 425°F. Spray a glass baking dish with nonstick cooking spray.

2. Fill each chili with chicken and cheese. Fold over the edges of the chilies and place them open side down in the dish.

3. In a medium bowl, whisk together egg substitute, eggs, flour, milk, salsa, and salt and pepper. Pour over the chilies.

4. Bake for 20 minutes. Remove from oven and sprinkle shredded cheddar cheese over the top. Return to the oven for 3–5 minutes more, until cheese is brown and bubbly. Cool before serving.

Exchanges
1 Starch
4 Very Lean Meat

Calories 238
  Calories from Fat . . 56
Total Fat . . . . 6 g
  Saturated Fat . . . . . . 4 g
Cholesterol . . . . 125 mg
Sodium . . . . 1418 mg
Carbohydrate . . . . . . 15 g
  Dietary Fiber . . . . . . 2 g
  Sugars . . . . 4 g
Protein . . . . 26 g

Multi-Bean and Turkey Salad with Feta Cheese

Serves 6   Serving size: 1 1/3 cups
Preparation time: 15 minutes
Standing time: 2 hours

DELI: smoked turkey

ALSO VISIT: shelves for beans, vinegar; salad bar or produce section for red onion, corn; produce for cilantro

- 1   14.5-oz can chickpeas, rinsed and drained
- 1   14.5-oz can black beans, rinsed and drained
- 1   14.5-oz can great northern beans, rinsed and drained
- 1   cup whole-kernel corn
- 2   cups diced smoked turkey (or use regular cooked turkey to reduce sodium)
- 1/4   cup finely chopped red onion
- 1/4   cup finely chopped cilantro (or parsley)
- 1/4   cup olive oil
- 3/4   cup balsamic vinegar
- 1/4   cup crumbled feta cheese
- 1   tsp black pepper
- 2   tsp sugar

1. Combine all ingredients in a large bowl.
2. Mix thoroughly but gently and refrigerate for at least 2 hours before serving.

Exchanges

3 Starch
2 Lean Meat
1/2 Monounsaturated Fat

Calories 385
  Calories from Fat . 111
Total Fat . . . . 12 g
  Saturated Fat . . . . . . 3 g
Cholesterol . . . . 26 mg
Sodium . . . . 1256 mg
Carbohydrate . . . . . . 49 g
  Dietary Fiber . . . . . 11 g
  Sugars . . . . 11 g
Protein . . . . 23 g

Barbecued Chicken Sandwich

Serves 4   Serving size: 1 bun, 1/2 cup filling
Preparation time: 5 minutes
Cooking time: 20 minutes

DELI: chicken breasts

ALSO VISIT: shelves for vinegar, ketchup, Worcestershire sauce; bakery section for whole-wheat buns

> 1/2 cup apple cider vinegar
>
> 2/3 cup ketchup
>
>   1 Tbsp Worcestershire sauce
>
>   2 tsp lemon juice
>
>   Hot sauce to taste
>
>   Pepper to taste
>
>   4 whole-wheat buns, sliced in half and toasted
>
>   2 cups roasted deli chicken breast, shredded (or use plain roasted chicken to reduce sodium)

1. In a medium saucepan, combine vinegar, ketchup, Worcestershire sauce, lemon juice, hot sauce, and pepper.

2. Bring to a boil and reduce heat. Simmer uncovered, stirring occasionally, until the sauce thickens, about 15 minutes.

3. Add the chicken and cook another 5 minutes. Remove from heat; let cool for about 5 minutes before serving.

4. Serve on buns either open-faced or as sandwiches.

Exchanges

2 Starch
1 Vegetable
2 Very Lean Meat

Calories 237
  Calories from Fat . . 29
Total Fat . . . . 3 g
  Saturated Fat . . . . . . 0 g
Cholesterol . . . . 25 mg
Sodium . . . . 1340 mg
Carbohydrate . . . . . . 36 g
  Dietary Fiber . . . . . . 2 g
  Sugars . . . . 9 g
Protein . . . . 18 g

Turkey Chili Potpie

Serves 6   Serving size: 2 cups
Preparation time: 15 minutes
Cooking time: 30 minutes

DELI: smoked turkey

ALSO VISIT: salad bar or produce section for red pepper, onion, corn; produce for garlic, cilantro; shelves for tomatoes, black beans, corn bread mix, chili spice mix

- 1 Tbsp olive oil
- 1 red bell pepper, cut into small pieces (1 1/2 cups)
- 2 Tbsp chopped garlic
- 1 large onion, chopped (1 1/2 cups)
- 2 cups diced smoked turkey (or use regular cooked turkey to reduce sodium)
- 1 package dried chili spice mix (or use 1 Tbsp chili powder to lower sodium content)
- 1 cup whole-kernel corn
- 1/4 cup finely chopped cilantro
- 1 20-oz can whole, peeled tomatoes in their own juices, coarsely chopped
- 1 14.5-oz can black beans, rinsed and drained

  Nonstick cooking spray
- 1 package (8.5 oz) corn bread mix (usually need 1 egg and water or milk to make)

1. Preheat oven to 400°F.

2. Heat the oil in a large skillet. Add the bell pepper, garlic, onion, turkey, and chili mix. Cook and stir for about 5–8 minutes, until the onions are translucent.

3. Stir in the corn and cilantro and cook another 2 minutes, stirring constantly. Add the tomatoes and their juices along with the beans and continue to stir until boiling. Remove from heat.

Exchanges
4 Starch
1 Very Lean Meat

Calories 348
  Calories from Fat . . 65
Total Fat . . . . 7 g
  Saturated Fat . . . . . . 3 g
Cholesterol . . . . 61 mg
Sodium . . . . 1402 mg
Carbohydrate . . . . . . 61 g
  Dietary Fiber . . . . . . 8 g
  Sugars . . . . 18 g
Protein . . . . 20 g

4. Spray the glass baking dish with nonstick spray and spoon the mixture into the baking dish.

5. In a separate bowl, mix the corn bread as instructed on the box. Spoon the corn bread over the top of the meat mixture. Bake for about 20–25 minutes, until the corn bread is golden brown. Let sit for 8–10 minutes before serving.

Creamy Parmesan-Basil Ham and Penne

Serves 4   Serving size: about 1 1/4 cups
Preparation time: 15 minutes
Cooking time: 10 minutes

DELI: ham, Parmesan cheese

ALSO VISIT: shelves for pasta, flour, spices; frozen foods for peas; dairy case for sour cream

8	oz uncooked penne pasta
1/2	cup frozen peas
2	tsp olive oil
2	cloves garlic, minced
1/4	lb ham slices, cut into bite-sized strips
1	8-oz container light sour cream
1/2	cup shredded fresh Parmesan cheese
3/4	cup fat-free milk
1	Tbsp flour
1	Tbsp fresh basil or 3/4 tsp dry

1. Prepare pasta according to package directions, adding peas during last 2 minutes. Drain and keep warm.

2. Meanwhile, in a large nonstick skillet, heat oil and garlic over medium heat 1–2 minutes or until garlic is light golden brown. Add ham; cook and stir for 1 minute.

3. In a small bowl, blend sour cream, Parmesan cheese, milk, and flour. Stir into ham mixture. Cook and stir until bubbly and slightly thickened. Reduce heat to low.

4. Add pasta and basil; toss to coat. Cook until thoroughly heated.

Exchanges
3 1/2 Starch
2 Lean Meat
1/2 Fat

Calories 408
  Calories from Fat . 111
Total Fat . . . . 12 g
  Saturated Fat . . . . . . 5 g
Cholesterol . . . . 37 mg
Sodium . . . . 530 mg
Carbohydrate . . . . . . 53 g
  Dietary Fiber . . . . . . 3 g
  Sugars . . . . 8 g
Protein . . . . 22 g

Fruited Chicken Salad

Serves 4   Serving size: 1 cup pasta, 1/2 cup chicken, about 1/2 cup fruit

Preparation time: 15 minutes

Cooking time: 12 minutes (for cooking pasta if not prepared before starting recipe)

DELI: chicken

ALSO VISIT: salad bar for pineapple, grapes, cantaloupe; dairy case for sour cream; shelves for pasta

> 4   cups cooked bow tie pasta (about 8 oz dry), cooled
>
> 2   cups diced cooked deli chicken
>
> 1/2   cup diced fresh pineapple
>
> 1/2   cup seedless red grapes, halved
>
> 1/2   cup diced cantaloupe
>
> 1   cup fat-free sour cream
>
> Romaine lettuce leaves (optional)

Combine all ingredients. Mix well. Serve immediately or refrigerate until serving. Serve on lettuce-lined plates if desired.

Exchanges

3 1/2 Starch
1/2 Fruit
3 Very Lean Meat

Calories 417
  Calories from Fat . . 59
Total Fat . . . . 7 g
  Saturated Fat . . . . . . 2 g
Cholesterol . . . . 67 mg
Sodium . . . . 664 mg
Carbohydrate . . . . . . 57 g
  Dietary Fiber . . . . . . 2 g
  Sugars . . . . 13 g
Protein . . . . 30 g

Ham and Vegetable Dinner Wraps

Serves 4   Serving size: 1/4 cup rice, 1 oz ham, 1/2 cup vegetables, 1 tortilla

Preparation time: 15 minutes

Cooking time: 20 minutes

DELI: ham, marinated vegetable salad

ALSO VISIT: produce for tomato; refrigerated section for tortillas; shelves for rice

- 1/2 cup uncooked instant white or brown rice
- 4 oz ham slices, cut into strips
- 1 cup deli marinated vegetable salad (drain most of oil)
- 1 tomato, chopped
- 4 10-inch fat-free tortillas (large), heated if desired

1. Prepare rice according to package directions, omitting salt and butter.

2. Heat a large nonstick skillet over medium heat. Add ham slices and marinated vegetables. Cook and stir for 5 minutes or until vegetables are tender-crisp. Stir in tomato. Heat through. Stir in rice and remove from heat.

3. Place 1/4 (about 3/4 cup) of ham mixture on each tortilla. Roll up and eat.

Exchanges

3 Starch
1 Vegetable
1 Very Lean Meat

Calories 277
   Calories from Fat . . 36
Total Fat . . . . 4 g
   Saturated Fat . . . . . . 1 g
Cholesterol . . . . 16 mg
Sodium . . . . 862 mg
Carbohydrate . . . . . . 50 g
   Dietary Fiber . . . . . . 3 g
   Sugars . . . . 3 g
Protein . . . . 13 g

Mediterranean Chicken and Pasta

Serves 4   Serving size: 1 cup pasta, 2 oz chicken, 3/4 cup spinach, 2 Tbsp cheese

Preparation time: 10 minutes

Cooking time: 15 minutes (includes cooking pasta if not already prepared)

DELI: chicken

ALSO VISIT: salad bar for spinach, feta cheese, onion; shelves for spices, broth

- 2 tsp olive oil
- 1 small onion, cut into thin wedges
- 2 cloves garlic, minced
- 8 oz cooked deli chicken breast, cut into 1/2-inch chunks
- 3/4 tsp dried oregano leaves
- 1/4 tsp crushed red pepper flakes
- 1/2 cup low-sodium, low-fat chicken broth
- 1 tsp grated lemon peel
- 3 cups sliced fresh spinach leaves
- 4 cups cooked pasta (any shape)
- 1/2 cup crumbled feta cheese

1. In a large nonstick skillet over medium-high heat, heat olive oil. Add garlic and onion. Cover and cook for 2 minutes.

2. Add chicken, oregano, and red pepper flakes. Cook and stir 1 minute or until chicken is hot. Stir in broth; bring to boil. Stir in lemon peel.

3. Add spinach; cook and stir 1 minute or just until spinach is wilted. Add pasta; toss to mix. Cook until heated through; then remove from heat.

4. Add feta and toss to mix.

Exchanges

3 Starch
2 Very Lean Meat

Calories 321
  Calories from Fat . . 63
Total Fat . . . . 7 g
  Saturated Fat . . . . . . 3 g
Cholesterol . . . . 33 mg
Sodium . . . . 709 mg
Carbohydrate . . . . . . 44 g
  Dietary Fiber . . . . . . 3 g
  Sugars . . . . 5 g
Protein . . . . 21 g

Portobello Beef Potatoes

Serves 4   Serving size: 1 potato, 1 oz beef
Preparation time: 15 minutes
Cooking time: 22 minutes (if potatoes are microwaved), 52 minutes (if potatoes are baked in the oven)

DELI: roast beef

ALSO VISIT: produce for potatoes, mushrooms, marjoram; salad bar for carrots, celery; shelves for gravy, wine; dairy for sour cream

- 4 small baking potatoes
- 2 shallots, thinly sliced
- 4 portobello mushroom caps, sliced
- 2/3 cup sliced baby carrot (or chopped carrot)
- 1/4 cup chopped celery
- 1 Tbsp chopped fresh marjoram (or 1/2 tsp dried)
- 1 clove garlic, minced
- 1/2 cup prepared fat-free beef gravy
- 2 Tbsp red wine or water
- 4 oz sliced cooked deli roast beef, cut into strips (about 1 cup)
- 1/3 cup fat-free sour cream (optional)

1. Microwave or bake potatoes until tender.

2. Meanwhile, spray medium nonstick skillet with nonstick cooking spray. Heat over medium heat. Add shallots, mushrooms, carrots, celery, marjoram, and garlic.

3. Add 2 Tbsp water, and cook, covered, 5–7 minutes or until carrots and mushrooms are tender.

4. Stir in gravy, wine or water, and beef. Cook until thoroughly heated. If desired, stir in 1/3 cup fat-free sour cream, heat thoroughly. Serve over split baked potatoes.

Exchanges
1 1/2 Starch
1 Vegetable
1 Very Lean Meat

Calories 187
  Calories from Fat . . 14
Total Fat . . . . 2 g
  Saturated Fat . . . . . . 1 g
Cholesterol . . . . 18 mg
Sodium . . . . 329 mg
Carbohydrate . . . . . . 31 g
  Dietary Fiber . . . . . . 4 g
  Sugars . . . . 4 g
Protein . . . . 12 g

Roast Beef Salad Pizza

Serves 4   Serving size: 1 pita, 2 oz beef, 1 oz cheese
Preparation time: 15 minutes
Cooking time: 5 minutes

DELI: roast beef, roasted red bell pepper strips

ALSO VISIT: bread department for pita; salad bar for broccoli, cauliflower; dairy case for cheese

- 4   6-inch whole-wheat pita breads
- 1/2 cup 50% reduced-fat garlic and herb spreadable cheese
- 1/2 lb thinly sliced cooked deli roast beef, cut into strips (about 1 cup)
- 1/3 cup roasted red bell pepper strips
- 3/4 cup broccoli florets
- 1/2 cup small cauliflower florets

1. Preheat oven to 350°F.

2. Wrap the pita breads in foil, place on a cookie sheet, and bake for 5 minutes. Remove from oven and cool for 1 minute.

3. Spread cheese evenly over each pita. Top with roast beef, red bell pepper, and broccoli and cauliflower florets. Cut in half to serve.

Exchanges
2 1/2 Starch
3 Very Lean Meat
1/2 Fat

Calories 320
  Calories from Fat . . 69
Total Fat . . . . 8 g
  Saturated Fat . . . . . . 3 g
Cholesterol . . . . 56 mg
Sodium . . . . 940 mg
Carbohydrate . . . . . . 38 g
  Dietary Fiber . . . . . . 3 g
  Sugars . . . . 7 g
Protein . . . . 27 g

Roasted Chicken Salad with Napa Cabbage

**Serves 4   Serving size: 4 oz chicken, 1 cup cabbage,
1/4 cup snow peas**
Preparation time: 10 minutes
Cooking time: 2 minutes

DELI: chicken

ALSO VISIT: produce for snow pea pods, carrots, Napa cabbage, garlic;
shelves for dressing

1 lb roasted white-meat deli chicken (either pulled from
a whole chicken and skinned or from sliced chicken),
cubed or shredded

1 cup fresh snow pea pods, halved

1/2 cup julienne baby carrot strips

1 clove garlic, minced

1/2 cup low-fat Oriental salad dressing or low-fat
vinaigrette

4 cups shredded Napa cabbage

1. In a large nonstick skillet over medium heat, heat the chicken, snow pea pods, carrots, and garlic. Cover and cook for 2 minutes. Stir in dressing. Remove from heat.

2. In a large bowl, combine the cabbage and chicken mixture; toss together until mixed.

Exchanges

1/2 Carbohydrate
4 Lean Meat
1/2 Fat

Calories	285
Calories from Fat	. 117
Total Fat	13 g
Saturated Fat	2 g
Cholesterol	100 mg
Sodium	416 mg
Carbohydrate	7 g
Dietary Fiber	1 g
Sugars	4 g
Protein	34 g

Roasted Red Pepper Turkey with Vermicelli

Serves 4   Serving size: 4 oz turkey, 1/2 cup pasta
Preparation time: 10 minutes
Cooking time: 5 minutes

DELI: turkey, roasted red pepper

ALSO VISIT: shelves for flour, broth, vermicelli noodles; produce for basil

> 3/4 cup roasted red bell pepper strips, drained
>
> 1/2 cup low-fat, low-sodium chicken broth
>
> 2 tsp flour
>
> 1/2 tsp sugar
>
> 1 lb cooked deli turkey breast, cut in 1/2-inch strips (or use plain cooked turkey to reduce sodium)
>
> 1 clove garlic, slivered
>
> 2 Tbsp thinly sliced fresh basil strips
>
> 2 cups cooked vermicelli noodles (4 oz uncooked)
>
> Parsley (optional)

1. In a blender or food processor, combine roasted pepper, broth, flour, and sugar; process until blended.

2. Spray a large skillet with nonstick cooking spray, and heat over medium-high heat. Add turkey and garlic; cook and stir for 1–2 minutes or until garlic is softened.

3. Add red pepper mixture. Reduce heat to medium. Cook, uncovered, until bubbly, stirring constantly. Stir in basil, and cook for 1 minute.

4. Serve over hot cooked pasta. Sprinkle with parsley, if desired.

Exchanges

3 Starch
3 Very Lean Meat

Calories	338
Calories from Fat	39
Total Fat	4 g
Saturated Fat	1 g
Cholesterol	52 mg
Sodium	1109 mg
Carbohydrate	47 g
Dietary Fiber	3 g
Sugars	5 g
Protein	32 g

Turkey with Leeks and Mushrooms

Serves 4   Serving size: 4 oz turkey
Preparation time: 10 minutes
Cooking time: 15 minutes

DELI: turkey

ALSO VISIT: produce for leeks, mushrooms; shelves for wine, flour; dairy case for sour cream

> 1   leek, halved lengthwise and sliced
> 1   cup sliced mushrooms
> 1/4   cup white wine
> 1   Tbsp fresh thyme leaves (or 1/4 tsp dry)
> 1   tsp flour
> 1/2   cup fat-free sour cream
> Dash white pepper
> 4   4-oz slices cooked deli turkey breast

1. In large nonstick skillet, combine leek, mushrooms, wine, and thyme. Cook, covered, over low to medium heat for 5–8 minutes or until leek is tender.

2. Stir flour into sour cream. Add sour cream mixture and pepper to skillet. Cook over medium heat until thoroughly heated.

3. Add turkey slices to skillet, spooning mushroom mixture over the top. Cover. Cook over low heat for 5 minutes to blend flavors.

Exchanges
1/2 Carbohydrate
4 Very Lean Meat

Calories 166
  Calories from Fat . . 30
Total Fat . . . . 3 g
  Saturated Fat . . . . . . 1 g
Cholesterol . . . . 54 mg
Sodium . . . . 1000 mg
Carbohydrate . . . . 8 g
  Dietary Fiber . . . . . . 1 g
  Sugars . . . . 3 g
Protein . . . . 26 g

Barbecued Chicken Salad

Serves 4 Serving size: 4 oz chicken, 1/2 cup vegetables, 1/4 cup beans
Preparation time: about 15 minutes
Cooking time: about 25 minutes

DELI: cooked chicken

ALSO VISIT: shelves for roasted red bell peppers, ketchup, sugar, vinegar, Worcestershire sauce, spices; salad bar for red onion, lettuce; frozen foods for corn

Barbecue Sauce:
- 1 cup ketchup (use low-sodium variety to reduce sodium)
- 2 Tbsp brown sugar
- 2 Tbsp red wine vinegar
- 1 cup water
- 2 Tbsp Worcestershire sauce
- 1–2 tsp cayenne pepper
- 2 tsp paprika
- 1 Tbsp canola oil

Salad:
- 1 cup diced roasted red bell peppers
- 1 cup frozen corn, thawed
- Fresh ground pepper to taste
- 1/2 medium diced red onion
- 1 lb diced cooked white-meat deli chicken
- 1 cup black beans, drained and rinsed
- 4 cups any dark lettuce

Exchanges

3 Starch
1 Vegetable
3 Very Lean Meat

Calories	349
Calories from Fat	53
Total Fat	6 g
Saturated Fat	0 g
Cholesterol	40 mg
Sodium	1942 mg
Carbohydrate	51 g
Dietary Fiber	8 g
Sugars	21 g
Protein	30 g

1. In a small saucepan, combine the barbecue sauce ingredients. Bring to a boil. Reduce heat and cook for 20 minutes until sauce is reduced by half.

2. Combine all salad ingredients.

3. Pour sauce over the salad. Serve at room temperature or chilled over lettuce.

Mexican Roll-Ups

Serves 6   Serving size: 4 oz roast beef, 1 12-inch tortilla
Preparation time: 15 minutes

DELI: roast beef

ALSO VISIT: salad bar for peppers, lettuce; refrigerated section for tortillas; shelves for vinegar, spices

> 6 12-inch flour tortillas (whole-wheat if available)
> 6 large romaine lettuce leaves
> 1 1/2 lb thinly sliced cooked deli roast beef
> 1 cup diced tomatoes
> 1 cup diced red and yellow bell peppers
> 2 Tbsp olive oil
> 3 Tbsp red wine vinegar
> 2 tsp cumin

1. For each roll-up, tear a 15-inch piece of either waxed paper or foil. Place the tortilla flat on the paper or foil. Place a romaine lettuce leaf on top of each tortilla. Divide the beef onto the lettuce leaves. Divide the tomatoes, peppers, oil, vinegar, and cumin over the beef.

2. Begin rolling the paper or foil over the tortilla to encase the filling. Roll until the sandwich is completely rolled up. Fold the excess paper or foil over the top and bottom of each roll-up. To eat, peel back the paper and foil.

Exchanges

2 Starch
1 Vegetable
4 Very Lean Meat
2 Monounsaturated Fat

Calories 425
  Calories from Fat . 132
Total Fat . . . . 15 g
  Saturated Fat . . . . . . 4 g
Cholesterol . . . . 72 mg
Sodium . . . . 939 mg
Carbohydrate . . . . . . 34 g
  Dietary Fiber . . . . . . 3 g
  Sugars . . . . 3 g
Protein . . . . 36 g

Chicken with Tomato Rosemary Sauce

Serves 4   Serving size: 3–4 oz chicken, 1/2 cup pasta, about 1 cup sauce

Preparation time: 20 minutes

Cooking time: 30 minutes

DELI: cooked chicken

ALSO VISIT: salad bar for onion, carrots; shelves for crushed tomatoes, olives, capers, wine, spices; produce for parsley

1/4	cup dry white wine
3	cloves garlic, minced
1	medium onion, diced
1	cup diced carrots
1	28-oz can crushed tomatoes
1	lb cooked deli chicken breast
2	tsp sugar
2	tsp dried rosemary, crumbled
1/2	cup minced Italian parsley
1/4	cup sliced black olives
2	tsp capers
	Fresh ground pepper and salt to taste
2	cups cooked pasta

Garnish: 2 Tbsp Parmesan cheese

1. Bring the wine to a boil in a heavy skillet over medium heat. Add the garlic and onion and sauté for 5 minutes. Add the carrots and sauté for 5 minutes more. Add the tomatoes and sugar.

2. Add the chicken to the skillet. Simmer, uncovered, for 10 minutes. Add the rosemary, parsley, olives, and capers. Simmer for 10 more minutes. Spoon over the pasta and sprinkle with Parmesan cheese before serving.

Exchanges

2 1/2 Starch
2 Vegetable
3 Very Lean Meat

Calories	363
Calories from Fat	52
Total Fat	6 g
Saturated Fat	1 g
Cholesterol	44 mg
Sodium	1681 mg
Carbohydrate	48 g
Dietary Fiber	8 g
Sugars	19 g
Protein	31 g

Chicken and Almond Stew

Serves 4   Serving size: 1 cup (4 oz chicken, 1/3 cup beans)
Preparation time: 20 minutes
Cooking time: 45 minutes

DELI: cooked chicken

ALSO VISIT: shelves for broth, almonds, beans, tomatoes, spices; salad bar for onion

- 1 Tbsp olive oil
- 1/2 cup chopped onion
- 2 cups low-fat, low-sodium chicken broth
- 1 cup diced canned tomatoes, drained
- 2 Tbsp slivered almonds
- 1 tsp chili powder
- 1/4 tsp cayenne pepper
- 1/2 tsp cinnamon
- 1 lb cubed cooked deli chicken
- 1 15-oz can black beans, rinsed and drained

1. In a large stockpot over medium-high heat, heat the oil. Add the onion and sauté for 3–5 minutes, stirring occasionally.

2. Add the broth, tomatoes, almonds, and spices. Bring to a boil, lower the heat, and simmer for 30 minutes.

3. Add the chicken and beans and simmer for 10 more minutes.

Exchanges

1 Starch
1 Vegetable
4 Very Lean Meat
1 Monounsaturated Fat

Calories	276
Calories from Fat	65
Total Fat	7 g
Saturated Fat	1 g
Cholesterol	40 mg
Sodium	1435 mg
Carbohydrate	25 g
Dietary Fiber	8 g
Sugars	8 g
Protein	31 g

White Bean and Turkey Soup

Serves 6   Serving size: 1 cup, 2 oz turkey
Preparation time: 15 minutes
Cooking time: about 50 minutes

DELI: cooked turkey breast

ALSO VISIT: shelves for broth, beans, spices; salad bar for celery, carrots, onion

1	Tbsp canola oil
1	medium onion, minced
3	medium carrots, diced
3	stalks celery, sliced
3	cups low-sodium, low-fat chicken broth
2	15-oz cans white beans, one can drained
1 1/4	cups diced cooked deli turkey
2	tsp paprika
1	tsp minced thyme
	Fresh ground pepper to taste

1. In a stockpot, heat the oil over medium-high heat. Add the onion and sauté for 5 minutes, stirring occasionally. Add the carrots and sauté for another 5 minutes. Add the celery and sauté for 2 minutes.

2. Add the broth and bring to a boil. Simmer over low heat for 5 minutes.

3. In a blender or food processor, puree one can of the beans with its liquid. Add to the soup. Simmer for 10 minutes.

4. Add the other can of whole beans, turkey, paprika, thyme, and pepper. Continue to simmer for 20 minutes.

Exchanges

2 Starch
1 Vegetable
1 Lean Meat

Calories 237
  Calories from Fat . . 34
Total Fat . . . . 4 g
  Saturated Fat . . . . . . 0 g
Cholesterol . . . . 14 mg
Sodium . . . . 890 mg
Carbohydrate . . . . . . 34 g
  Dietary Fiber . . . . . . 8 g
  Sugars . . . . 6 g
Protein . . . . 18 g

Quick Hoppin' John

Serves 6   Serving size: 1 cup
Preparation time: 20 minutes
Cooking time: 35 minutes

DELI: smoked turkey

ALSO VISIT: salad bar for onion, carrots, celery; shelves for peas, broth; frozen foods for collard greens

1	Tbsp canola oil
1	medium onion, chopped
1/2	cup diced carrots
1/2	cup diced celery
2	cloves garlic, minced
2	15-oz cans black-eyed peas, drained
1	tsp minced fresh thyme
2	10-oz pkg frozen collard greens, slightly thawed
1	cup white rice
2 1/2	cups low-fat, low-sodium chicken broth
1	cup diced smoked turkey breast (or use regular diced cooked turkey to reduce sodium)
	Fresh ground pepper to taste

1. In a stockpot, heat the oil over medium heat. Add the onion and carrots and sauté for 5 minutes. Add the celery and garlic and sauté for 3 more minutes.

2. Add the black-eyed peas, thyme, collard greens, and rice. Sauté for 2 minutes. Add the chicken broth. Bring to a boil. Lower the heat, cover, and cook for 20 minutes, until water is absorbed and rice is tender.

3. Add the turkey and cook 5 more minutes. Sprinkle with fresh ground pepper to taste.

Exchanges
3 Starch
2 Vegetable
1 Very Lean Meat

Calories 319
  Calories from Fat . . 32
Total Fat . . . . 4 g
  Saturated Fat . . . . . . 0 g
Cholesterol . . . . 11 mg
Sodium . . . . 690 mg
Carbohydrate . . . . . . 54 g
  Dietary Fiber . . . . . 10 g
  Sugars . . . . 5 g
Protein . . . . 18 g

Real Barbecued Roast Beef Open-Faced Sandwiches

Serves 4   Serving size: 3–4 oz meat, 1 slice bread, 1 tomato slice
Preparation time: 10 minutes
Marinating time: 1 hour

DELI: lean roast beef

ALSO VISIT: salad bar for onions; shelves for spices, lemon juice; bakery department for rye bread; produce for tomato

Barbecue marinade:
- 1 Tbsp chili powder
- 1 tsp ground ginger
- 2 cloves garlic, minced
- 1 small onion, minced
- 1/3 cup lemon juice
- 2 Tbsp olive oil
- 2 tsp paprika

Sandwich:
- 1 lb sliced cooked deli roast beef
- 4 slices rye bread, toasted
- 4 slices tomato

1. Combine the barbecue marinade with the roast beef and marinate for 1 hour.

2. Drain marinade from roast beef and divide roast beef equally among the slices of rye bread.

3. Top with tomato slices and serve.

Exchanges

1 Starch
4 Very Lean Meat
1 Monounsaturated Fat

Calories	293
Calories from Fat	78
Total Fat	9 g
Saturated Fat	3 g
Cholesterol	72 mg
Sodium	741 mg
Carbohydrate	18 g
Dietary Fiber	2 g
Sugars	2 g
Protein	33 g

Turkey and Cranberry Salad

**Serves 4   Serving size: 1 cup turkey, 1/4 cup fruit and veggies
Preparation time: 17 minutes**

DELI: cooked turkey

ALSO VISIT: shelves for cranberries, vinegar; salad bar for red onion,
yellow bell pepper, green onions; produce for parsley

Salad:
4 cups diced cooked deli turkey

1/2 cup rehydrated cranberries, drained (to rehydrate dried
cranberries, pour boiling water over 1/2 cup cranberries
and let sit for 10 minutes)

1/4 cup diced red onion

1/4 cup diced yellow bell pepper

Dressing:
1/2 cup raspberry vinegar

2 Tbsp olive oil

2 Tbsp minced parsley

1 Tbsp minced green onions

Fresh ground pepper to taste

1. Combine all salad ingredients in a large
bowl.

2. Mix dressing ingredients in a blender.
Pour the dressing over the salad and toss
well. Serve at room temperature.

Exchanges

1 Fruit
4 Lean Meat

Calories 271
Calories from Fat . . 98
Total Fat . . . . 11 g
Saturated Fat . . . . . . 1 g
Cholesterol . . . . 64 mg
Sodium . . . . 1184 mg
Carbohydrate . . . . . . 15 g
Dietary Fiber . . . . . . 2 g
Sugars . . . . 12 g
Protein . . . . 30 g

Italian Turkey Sauté

Serves 4 Serving size: 3–4 oz turkey with sauce
Preparation time: 15 minutes
Cooking time: 20 minutes

DELI: turkey

ALSO VISIT: shelves for crushed tomatoes, red wine, capers; salad bar for onions; produce for garlic, fresh herbs

2	tsp olive oil
1/2	cup diced onion
2	cloves garlic, minced
1 1/2	cups crushed tomatoes
2	Tbsp red wine
2	tsp minced fresh oregano
1	lb cubed cooked deli turkey (preferably white meat)
2	Tbsp minced fresh basil
2	Tbsp capers

1. In a large skillet over medium-high heat, heat the oil. Add the onion and sauté for 3 minutes. Add the garlic and sauté for 2 minutes, stirring occasionally.

2. Add the crushed tomatoes and wine. Bring to a boil. Lower the heat and simmer for 10 minutes. Add the remaining ingredients and heat thoroughly.

Exchanges
2 Vegetable
3 Very Lean Meat
1/2 Fat

Calories 192
    Calories from Fat . . 51
Total Fat . . . . 6 g
    Saturated Fat . . . . . . 2 g
Cholesterol . . . . 52 mg
Sodium . . . . 1344 mg
Carbohydrate . . . . . . 10 g
    Dietary Fiber . . . . . . 3 g
    Sugars . . . . 6 g
Protein . . . . 26 g

Sun-Dried Tomato Turkey Salad

Serves 4   Serving size: 3–4 oz turkey, about 1 cup vegetables
Preparation time: 20 minutes

DELI: turkey

ALSO VISIT: salad bar for zucchini, celery, green onions, carrots; shelves for mayonnaise, sun-dried tomatoes, pesto

- 1 lb deli turkey, sliced 1 inch thick and cubed
- 1 cup sliced zucchini
- 1 cup sliced celery
- 1/2 cup sliced green onions
- 1/2 cup sliced carrots
- 3/4 cup low-fat mayonnaise
- 1/2 cup rehydrated sun-dried tomatoes, sliced
- 1 tsp prepared pesto
- Salt and fresh ground pepper to taste

1. In a salad bowl, combine the turkey, zucchini, celery, green onions, and carrots. Toss to mix.

2. In a small bowl, combine the mayonnaise, sun-dried tomatoes, and pesto. Season with salt and pepper.

3. Add the mayonnaise mixture to the turkey and mix well. Refrigerate for 1 hour before serving.

Exchanges

1 Carbohydrate
1 Vegetable
3 Very Lean Meat
1/2 Polyunsaturated Fat

Calories	235
Calories from Fat	62
Total Fat	7 g
Saturated Fat	1 g
Cholesterol	52 mg
Sodium	1431 mg
Carbohydrate	20 g
Dietary Fiber	3 g
Sugars	13 g
Protein	26 g

Smoked Turkey and Rice Soup

Serves 4   Serving size: 3 oz turkey, 1/4 cup rice, 1 cup broth
Preparation time: 20 minutes
Cooking time: 30 minutes

DELI: smoked turkey

ALSO VISIT: shelves for broth, rice; produce for onion, garlic, carrot

2	tsp olive oil
1	medium onion, diced
2	cloves garlic, minced
1	medium carrot, diced
1/4	tsp turmeric
	Dash ground red pepper
4 1/2	cups low-fat, low-sodium chicken broth
1	cup cooked white rice
12	oz cooked smoked deli turkey, sliced 1/2 inch thick and cubed
	Fresh ground pepper to taste

1. In a stockpot over medium heat, heat the oil. Add the onion and garlic and sauté for 3 minutes. Add the carrot and sauté for 4 minutes.

2. Add the turmeric and ground red pepper. Cook for 1 minute.

3. Add the broth and simmer the mixture over low heat for 10 minutes.

4. Add the rice and turkey. Season with pepper. Simmer for 15 more minutes.

Exchanges
1 Starch
3 Very Lean Meat

Calories 190
  Calories from Fat . . 30
Total Fat . . . . 3 g
  Saturated Fat . . . . . . 1 g
Cholesterol . . . . 39 mg
Sodium . . . . 1567 mg
Carbohydrate . . . . . . 17 g
  Dietary Fiber . . . . . . 1 g
  Sugars . . . . 4 g
Protein . . . . 22 g

*R*ecipes Using Frozen Foods

IN THIS SECTION YOU WILL BE ABLE TO USE FROZEN FOODS that you can purchase well in advance. The advantage of this, of course, is that you can simply look to your freezer whenever you want to prepare dinner. Frozen foods have come a long way since the days of TV dinners. Today there are a myriad of frozen foods that are healthy and can serve as a base for creative dinners.

A note about selection and storage of frozen foods. First, make sure that the food does not have a covering of ice crystals. This indicates the food has been thawed and refrozen. When you take the food home, be sure to label the package with the date of purchase. Generally, most frozen food is best used in three to six months. Rotate items so that old frozen food is used before new packages are used. Check the chart on page 10 for safe refrigerator and freezer storage times.

While some foods freeze well and with minimal preparation, others require special handling, and some should not be frozen at all. Do not freeze:

- Cooked egg whites and soft meringues

- Gelatin

- Cake or pie with custard filling

- Mayonnaise

- Cloves and imitation vanilla

- Milk, light cream, or sour cream

- Vegetables with high water content (celery, tomatoes, leafy salad greens, fennel, and so on, unless they have been cooked and finely chopped)

Here are some other helpful freezing tips.

- If you are going to thaw frozen foods, be sure to thaw only what you need. Do not place completely thawed foods back into the freezer.

- Before freezing fish, dip it in lemon juice to help preserve its original taste and texture. Then wrap it snugly in plastic wrap, followed by a layer of aluminum foil.

- A convenient way to freeze egg whites is in an ice cube tray, one per cube. When solid, transfer the frozen egg white cubes to freezer bags.

- Cheddar, Swiss, Gouda, mozzarella, and Parmesan cheeses freeze well but should be frozen in portions of no more than 2 pounds. Wrap the cheese tightly, first in plastic wrap, then aluminum foil, before freezing. Thaw in the refrigerator overnight to prevent crumbling.

- Fruits that freeze well include berries, citrus, figs, peaches, and cherries.

- In the frozen state, ginger is easier to peel and grate. Ginger keeps for several months.

- When you add items to your freezer, limit them to about 2 pounds for each cubic foot of freezer space.

Recipes

Stir-Fried Fajita Burritos

Serves 4   **Serving size: 1 burrito (1 tortilla, 3–4 oz chicken, 1 cup vegetables)**
Preparation time: 15 minutes
Cooking time: 10 minutes

FROZEN FOODS: burrito-size tortillas, peppers, onions

ALSO VISIT: deli for cooked chicken; salad bar for tomatoes, lettuce; shelves for taco seasoning; dairy case for cheese, sour cream

1	Tbsp canola oil
1	1-lb bag frozen peppers and onions
1	1-oz pkg taco seasoning mix
1	lb cooked chicken, cubed
4	burrito-size fat-free tortillas, warmed
1	cup diced, seeded tomatoes
1/2	cup reduced-fat shredded cheddar cheese
	Shredded lettuce
	Reduced-fat sour cream (optional)

1. In a wok over medium-high heat, heat the oil. Add the frozen peppers and onions and stir for 5 minutes until broken up. Add the taco seasoning and cook for 3–4 minutes.

2. Add the chicken and cook another 5 minutes, adding a little water or chicken broth if necessary to prevent burning. Remove from heat.

3. Spoon 1/4 of the mixture into the center of each tortilla and garnish with tomatoes, cheese, lettuce, and (if you wish) sour cream. Fold over the sides of the tortilla and roll up.

Exchanges
2 1/2 Starch
1 Vegetable
3 Very Lean Meat

Calories 338
  Calories from Fat . . 45
Total Fat . . . . 5 g
  Saturated Fat . . . . . . 0 g
Cholesterol . . . . 40 mg
Sodium . . . . 1861 mg
Carbohydrate . . . . . . 48 g
  Dietary Fiber . . . . . . 5 g
  Sugars . . . . 10 g
Protein . . . . 30 g

Creamy Chicken Bake

**Serves 4   Serving size: 2 chicken thighs, 1/2 cup vegetables,
1/2 cup rice**
Preparation time: 10 minutes
Cooking time: 1 hour

FROZEN FOODS: frozen vegetables

ALSO VISIT: meat department for chicken; shelves for soup, broth, herb mix, spices

8	skinless chicken thighs
1	Tbsp salt-free herb mix
1	tsp dried thyme leaves
1	tsp paprika
1	medium onion, chopped
1	8-oz pkg frozen mixed vegetables
1/2	10.75-oz can 98% fat-free cream of chicken soup
1/2	cup low-fat, low-sodium chicken broth
2	cups cooked brown rice

1. Preheat oven to 350°F.

2. Lay chicken thighs in a roasting pan and sprinkle with herbs. Add onion and frozen vegetables.

3. Stir together soup and broth and pour mixture over chicken and vegetables. Cover with roaster lid. Cook for 45 minutes to 1 hour or until chicken juices run clear.

4. Serve over rice.

Exchanges
2 Starch
1 Vegetable
4 Very Lean Meat
1/2 Fat

Calories 344
    Calories from Fat . . 65
Total Fat . . . . 7 g
    Saturated Fat . . . . . . 2 g
Cholesterol . . . . 117 mg
Sodium . . . . 366 mg
Carbohydrate . . . . . . 36 g
    Dietary Fiber . . . . . . 4 g
    Sugars . . . . 5 g
Protein . . . . 33 g

Quick Wonton Soup

Serves 4   Serving size: 1 1/2 cups
Preparation time: 5 minutes
Cooking time: 10 minutes

FROZEN FOODS: wontons or dumplings

ALSO VISIT: shelves for broth, spices, soy sauce; salad bar for green onions

6	cups low-fat, low-sodium chicken broth
8	frozen wontons or dumplings (reduced-fat)
1	tsp ground ginger
2	Tbsp lite soy sauce
1/4	cup minced green onion
	Hot sauce or spicy Chinese mustard to taste

1. Bring broth to a boil. Add wontons, ginger, soy sauce, and hot sauce or mustard.

2. Cook about 5 minutes or according to wonton/dumpling package directions, adding the green onions during the last 2 minutes.

Exchanges

1 Starch

Calories 76
   Calories from Fat . . . 6
Total Fat . . . . 1 g
   Saturated Fat . . . . . . 0 g
Cholesterol . . . . 0 mg
Sodium . . . . 1067 mg
Carbohydrate . . . . . . 10 g
   Dietary Fiber . . . . . . 0 g
   Sugars . . . . 4 g
Protein . . . . 6 g

Sweet and Sour Stir-Fried Cabbage and Dumplings

Serves 4   Serving size: 4 dumplings, 3/4 cup cabbage
Preparation time: 10 minutes
Cooking time: 8 minutes

FROZEN FOODS: dumplings

ALSO VISIT: shelves for spices, honey, oil, soy sauce, vinegar; produce for coleslaw mix

16	frozen vegetable dumplings (2 6.4-oz pkg), defrosted in refrigerator overnight or in microwave according to pkg directions
1 1/2	cups fat-free, reduced-sodium chicken broth
3	cups shredded cabbage and carrots (preshredded coleslaw mix)
1/2	cup sliced green onions
1/2	tsp ground ginger
1	tsp onion powder
1/2	Tbsp honey
1/2	Tbsp sesame oil
2	Tbsp lite soy sauce
2	Tbsp rice vinegar
1	Tbsp apple cider vinegar

1. Combine broth, cabbage and carrots, and green onion in a wok and stir-fry for 5 minutes.

2. Combine the ground ginger, onion powder, honey, sesame oil, soy sauce, rice vinegar, and apple cider vinegar. Add to the cabbage-carrot mixture. Add dumplings at end and cook until heated through.

Exchanges
1 Starch
1 Vegetable
1/2 Fat

Calories 125
  Calories from Fat . . 27
Total Fat . . . . 3 g
  Saturated Fat . . . . . . 1 g
Cholesterol . . . . 0 mg
Sodium . . . . 575 mg
Carbohydrate . . . . . . 21 g
  Dietary Fiber . . . . . . 2 g
  Sugars . . . . 9 g
Protein . . . . 4 g

Quick Fried Chicken Salad

**Serves 4   Serving size: 1–2 oz chicken, 1 cup salad,
2/3 cup vegetables, 2 Tbsp dressing, 2 Tbsp croutons**
Preparation time: 10 minutes
Cooking time: 10 minutes

FROZEN FOODS: chicken

ALSO VISIT: salad bar or produce section for cucumbers, tomatoes, mixed greens, green onions, feta; deli for roasted red pepper; shelves for dressing, croutons

2	pieces (4 oz each) frozen breaded and baked chicken breast
4	cups mixed salad greens
1	cup seeded and diced cucumbers
1	cup seeded and diced tomatoes
1/2	cup crumbled feta cheese
1/2	cup sliced roasted red pepper
1/2	cup fat-free croutons
1	Tbsp chopped green onions
1/2	cup fat-free honey-mustard salad dressing

1. Preheat oven to 400°F. Place the chicken breasts on a small cookie sheet. Bake until cooked through, about 10 minutes. Remove chicken from the oven and cut into strips. Set aside.

2. In a salad bowl, mix together salad greens, cucumbers, and tomatoes. In alternating strips across the greens, place the chicken, feta, and roasted red pepper. Sprinkle croutons and green onions on top. Drizzle with salad dressing before serving.

Exchanges

2 Starch
1 Vegetable
1 Lean Meat
1 Fat

Calories	279
Calories from Fat	80
Total Fat	9 g
Saturated Fat	3 g
Cholesterol	30 mg
Sodium	889 mg
Carbohydrate	33 g
Dietary Fiber	2 g
Sugars	9 g
Protein	14 g

Curried Shrimp and Butternut Squash Soup

Serves 4   Serving size: 1 cup
Preparation time: 10 minutes
Cooking time: 10 minutes

FROZEN FOODS: squash, shrimp

ALSO VISIT: shelves for evaporated fat-free milk, spices, coconut

2	8-oz pkg frozen pureed butternut squash (called "cooked squash" or "cooked winter squash")
1	12-oz can evaporated fat-free milk
2 tsp	sugar
1/2 tsp	pumpkin pie spice
8 oz	frozen, peeled medium shrimp (cooked or uncooked), rinsed under cold water for 2–3 minutes
1 Tbsp	curry powder
	Salt and fresh ground pepper to taste
2 tsp	flaked coconut

1. In a medium saucepan over medium-high heat, bring the squash and milk to a boil. Reduce heat to low and simmer for 5 minutes.

2. Add sugar and pumpkin pie spice and continue to simmer for 5 minutes more.

3. Add the shrimp, curry powder, salt, and pepper and cook 1 more minute. Add the coconut and serve.

4. Ladle the butternut squash soup into individual bowls with equal portions of the shrimp spooned on top.

Exchanges

1 Starch
1 Fat-Free Milk
1 Very Lean Meat

Calories 180
   Calories from Fat . . 10
Total Fat . . . . 1 g
   Saturated Fat . . . . . . 0 g
Cholesterol . . . . 95 mg
Sodium . . . . 233 mg
Carbohydrate . . . . . . 25 g
   Dietary Fiber . . . . . . 3 g
   Sugars . . . . 13 g
Protein . . . . 19 g

Sesame Ginger Fish

Serves 4   Serving size: 3–4 oz
Preparation time: 10 minutes
Cooking time: 10 minutes
Standing time: 30 minutes

FROZEN FOODS: fish

ALSO VISIT: shelves for spices, vinegar, soy sauce, sugar, sesame seeds; salad bar for green onions

> 4 4-oz pieces frozen fish (swordfish, salmon, catfish, etc.), defrosted in refrigerator overnight
>
> Marinade:
> 1 1/2 tsp ground ginger
> 2 tsp white pepper
> Salt and fresh ground pepper to taste
> 1/4 cup rice wine vinegar
> 1/4 cup lite soy sauce
> 1 1/2 tsp sesame seeds, toasted
> 1 tsp brown sugar
> 2 Tbsp minced green onions

1. Combine the marinade ingredients in a large bowl and whisk together. Add the fish, cover, and let marinate in the refrigerator for 30 minutes.

2. Preheat the oven to broil. Discard the marinade. Place the marinated fish on a nonstick broiler pan. Broil for a total of 8–10 minutes, turning once.

Exchanges
4 Very Lean Meat

Calories 143
  Calories from Fat . . 41
Total Fat . . . . 5 g
  Saturated Fat . . . . . . 0 g
Cholesterol . . . . 44 mg
Sodium . . . . 297 mg
Carbohydrate . . . . 1 g
  Dietary Fiber . . . . . . 0 g
  Sugars . . . . 1 g
Protein . . . . 23 g

Balsamic-Rosemary Chicken

Serves 4   Serving size: 3–4 oz
Preparation time: 10 minutes
Cooking time: 30 minutes
Standing time: 2–3 hours

FROZEN FOODS: chicken

ALSO VISIT: shelves for Dijon mustard, vinegar; produce for garlic and rosemary

- 4 4-oz pieces frozen boneless, skinless chicken breasts, defrosted in refrigerator overnight
- 2 Tbsp Dijon mustard
- Salt and fresh ground pepper to taste
- 2 Tbsp minced garlic
- 2 Tbsp water
- 1/4 cup white balsamic vinegar
- 4 sprigs fresh rosemary

1. Place chicken pieces in a casserole dish. Smooth mustard over chicken. Sprinkle with salt and pepper and garlic.

2. Pour water and vinegar over the chicken. Place one sprig of rosemary over each piece. Cover with foil and refrigerate for 2–3 hours to marinate.

3. Preheat the oven to 350°F. Place the covered casserole dish in the oven and bake for 20 minutes. Remove the foil and bake for 10 more minutes to brown the chicken.

Exchanges
1/2 Carbohydrate
3 Very Lean Meat

Calories 157
  Calories from Fat . . 28
Total Fat . . . . 3 g
  Saturated Fat . . . . . . 1 g
Cholesterol . . . . 68 mg
Sodium . . . . 156 mg
Carbohydrate . . . . 5 g
  Dietary Fiber . . . . . . 0 g
  Sugars . . . . 4 g
Protein . . . . 26 g

Corn and Three-Pepper Pudding

Serves 4   Serving size: 1 cup
Preparation time: 15 minutes
Cooking time: 45 minutes

FROZEN FOODS: corn, pepper medley, egg substitute

ALSO VISIT: shelves for evaporated fat-free milk, spices

1	10-oz pkg frozen corn
1/2	of 1-lb pkg frozen pepper stir-fry (3-pepper medley w/onions)
1	12-oz can evaporated fat-free milk
1	Tbsp butter, melted
	Salt and fresh ground pepper to taste
2	tsp sugar
1 1/2	tsp Italian seasoning
1/2	tsp paprika
1/2	cup egg substitute

1. Preheat oven to 350°F.

2. Defrost the frozen corn and peppers in the microwave. Chop peppers and onions into bite-size pieces.

3. Combine all ingredients and pour into a glass casserole dish that has been sprayed with nonstick spray. Bake for 45 minutes until center is set and firm.

Exchanges
1 1/2 Starch
1 Fat-Free Milk
1/2 Saturated Fat

Calories 207
  Calories from Fat . . 31
Total Fat . . . . 3 g
  Saturated Fat . . . . . . 2 g
Cholesterol . . . . 8 mg
Sodium . . . . 218 mg
Carbohydrate . . . . . . 33 g
  Dietary Fiber . . . . . . 3 g
  Sugars . . . . 15 g
Protein . . . . 13 g

Summer Shrimp Salad

Serves 4   Serving size: 3–4 oz shrimp
Preparation time: 15 minutes
Standing time: 1 hour

FROZEN FOODS: shrimp, peas

ALSO VISIT: salad bar for green onion, celery, tomato; shelves for spices, mayonnaise

1	lb frozen cooked medium shrimp
5	oz frozen peas
1/2	cup low-fat mayonnaise
2	Tbsp minced green onion
1/4	cup minced celery
1/4	cup chopped roasted red bell pepper
1	tsp garlic salt
1	tsp paprika
1	tsp black pepper
1/2	tsp cumin
1/2	tsp oregano
	Salt to taste
8	tomato wedges

1. Thaw the shrimp and peas thoroughly.

2. In a large bowl, mix the thawed shrimp and peas with the mayonnaise, celery, green onion, red bell pepper, and spices. Refrigerate for 1 hour. Serve with tomato wedges.

Exchanges
1 Carbohydrate
3 Very Lean Meat

Calories 188
  Calories from Fat . . 30
Total Fat . . . . 3 g
  Saturated Fat . . . . . . 0 g
Cholesterol . . . . 190 mg
Sodium . . . . 808 mg
Carbohydrate . . . . . . 16 g
  Dietary Fiber . . . . . . 3 g
  Sugars . . . . 10 g
Protein . . . . 23 g

Mexican Chicken Cutlets

Serves 4   Serving size: 4 oz
Preparation time: 10 minutes
Cooking time: 15 minutes

FROZEN FOODS: peppers and onions, chicken

ALSO VISIT: shelves for taco seasoning, broth

> 1   1-lb bag frozen peppers and onions
>
> 1   lb frozen boneless, skinless chicken cutlets, defrosted
>
> 1/2 pkg taco seasoning mix (use more or less depending on desired spiciness)
>
> 1/2 cup fat-free, reduced-sodium chicken broth

1. Combine all ingredients in a large nonstick skillet and bring to a boil over medium-high heat.

2. Lower the heat, cover, and simmer for 15 minutes. Add more broth if necessary.

Exchanges

1 Vegetable
4 Very Lean Meat

Calories	170
Calories from Fat	15
Total Fat	2 g
Saturated Fat	0 g
Cholesterol	64 mg
Sodium	383 mg
Carbohydrate	9 g
Dietary Fiber	2 g
Sugars	6 g
Protein	27 g

Sugar Snap Pea Stir-Fry with Chicken

Serves 4   Serving size: 3–4 oz chicken, 3/4 cup vegetables
Preparation time: 10 minutes
Cooking time: 15 minutes

FROZEN FOODS: sugar snap pea stir-fry mix

ALSO VISIT: shelves for sesame oil, water chestnuts, teriyaki sauce, sesame seeds; meat department for chicken (or purchase frozen chicken and defrost)

1	1-lb bag sugar snap pea stir-fry mix
1	Tbsp sesame oil
1	lb boneless, skinless chicken breasts, cut into 2-inch strips
1 1/2	cups shredded cabbage
1	8-oz can sliced water chestnuts, drained
1	cup lite teriyaki sauce, divided
2	Tbsp sesame seeds, toasted

1. Heat the sesame oil in a wok over medium-high heat. Add the chicken and cabbage. Cook for 3–5 minutes, stirring constantly.

2. Add the water chestnuts, vegetables, and 1 Tbsp of teriyaki sauce. Cover and cook for 5–7 minutes. Uncover, add remaining teriyaki sauce, and heat through. Sprinkle sesame seeds on top before serving.

Exchanges
2 Carbohydrate
4 Very Lean Meat
1/2 Fat

Calories 327
    Calories from Fat . . 78
Total Fat . . . . 9 g
    Saturated Fat . . . . . . 2 g
Cholesterol . . . . 68 mg
Sodium . . . . 1378 mg
Carbohydrate . . . . . . 26 g
    Dietary Fiber . . . . . . 4 g
    Sugars . . . . 19 g
Protein . . . . 32 g

Pierogie, Kielbasa, and Cabbage Casserole

Serves 4   Serving size: 4 oz sausage, 3 pierogies
Preparation time: 10 minutes
Cooking time: 30 minutes

FROZEN FOODS: pierogies

ALSO VISIT: meat department for sausage; produce for coleslaw mix, onion; shelves for chicken broth

1 lb reduced-fat Polish sausage, cut into 1/2-inch slices

Butter-flavored nonstick cooking spray

1 medium onion, thinly sliced

2 cups shredded coleslaw mix

12 frozen potato-and-onion pierogies, boiled 3–5 minutes to defrost

1 cup fat-free, reduced-sodium chicken broth, divided

1. Preheat oven to 350°F. Spray four individual casserole dishes with butter-flavored nonstick cooking spray.

2. Divide the onion and coleslaw mix between the casseroles. Divide the sausage among the casseroles. Top with 3 pierogies per casserole, and pour 1/4 cup chicken broth over each casserole.

3. Cover each casserole with foil. Bake covered for 20 minutes, then uncover and bake 10 minutes more.

Exchanges
3 Starch
2 Medium-Fat Meat

Calories 388
  Calories from Fat . 118
Total Fat . . . . 13 g
  Saturated Fat . . . . . . 5 g
Cholesterol . . . . 60 mg
Sodium . . . . 1524 mg
Carbohydrate . . . . . . 46 g
  Dietary Fiber . . . . . . 2 g
  Sugars . . . . 18 g
Protein . . . . 21 g

Spanish Fish

Serves 4   Serving size: 3–4 oz fish, 1/2 cup rice
Preparation time: 10 minutes
Cooking time: 35 minutes

FROZEN FOODS: fish, peas

ALSO VISIT: shelves for salsa, Spanish rice mix, stewed tomatoes

- 1 cup white rice
- 1 Tbsp olive oil
- 1 14.5-oz can stewed tomatoes, with juice
- 1 10-oz pkg frozen peas
- 4 4-oz frozen fish fillets (sole, flounder, perch, haddock, or cod), thawed
- 1 cup chunky salsa (mild, medium, or hot)

1. In a skillet that has a lid, sauté the rice in olive oil for 2 minutes. Add the stewed tomatoes.

2. Stir peas into the rice and tomatoes. Lay the fish fillets over this mixture.

3. Pour 1 cup of salsa over the top of the fish. Bring to a boil, then lower the heat. Cover and cook for 15–20 minutes over low heat until rice is cooked and fish is tender.

Exchanges

3 Starch
2 Vegetable
2 Very Lean Meat

Calories 384
  Calories from Fat . . 43
Total Fat . . . . 5 g
  Saturated Fat . . . . . . 1 g
Cholesterol . . . . 48 mg
Sodium . . . . 815 mg
Carbohydrate . . . . . . 58 g
  Dietary Fiber . . . . . . 5 g
  Sugars . . . . 10 g
Protein . . . . 28 g

Fish and Corn Chowder

Serves 4   Serving size: about 1 1/2 cups (3–4 oz fish)
Preparation time: 20 minutes
Cooking time: 15 minutes

FROZEN FOODS: corn, fish

ALSO VISIT: produce or salad bar for carrot, zucchini, celery, onion, dill, garlic; shelves for evaporated fat-free milk, flour; dairy case for milk

1 Tbsp olive oil

1 10-oz pkg frozen corn

3/4 cup chopped carrot

3/4 cup chopped zucchini

2 stalks celery, chopped

1 medium onion, chopped

2 cloves garlic, chopped

2 tsp fresh marjoram

2 tsp minced fresh dill

1/4 cup flour

1 lb frozen cod or white fish, defrosted and cut into 2-inch cubes

1 12-oz can evaporated fat-free milk

1 cup low-fat milk

2 cups water

Salt and fresh ground pepper to taste

Exchanges

1 1/2 Starch
1 Fat Free Milk
1 Vegetable
3 Very Lean Meat

Calories 338
    Calories from Fat . . 51
Total Fat . . . . 6 g
    Saturated Fat . . . . . . 1 g
Cholesterol . . . . 50 mg
Sodium . . . . 242 mg
Carbohydrate . . . . . . 40 g
    Dietary Fiber . . . . . . 4 g
    Sugars . . . . 16 g
Protein . . . . 33 g

1. In a large saucepot over medium-high heat, heat the olive oil.

2. Add the corn and sauté for 5 minutes, until the corn is defrosted. Add the carrot, zucchini, celery, onion, and garlic and sauté for 5 more minutes.

3. Add the marjoram and dill. Sauté for 2 minutes. Add the flour and stir to coat the vegetables.

4. Add the fish, evaporated skim milk, low-fat milk, and water. Bring to a simmer. Simmer for 5–10 minutes until slightly thickened. Season with salt and pepper.

Vegetable Couscous

Serves 4   Serving size: 1 cup
Preparation time: 20 minutes
Cooking time: 15 minutes (includes cooking couscous)

FROZEN FOODS: mixed vegetables, winter squash

ALSO VISIT: shelves for oil, broth, raisins, chickpeas, spices, couscous; produce for onion, garlic

1/2	of 1-lb bag mixed vegetables (any kind except w/water chestnuts), thawed
1	10-oz bag or box frozen cooked winter squash, thawed
2	Tbsp olive oil
1	large onion, diced
1	clove garlic, minced
1	cup low-fat, low-sodium chicken broth
1/4	cup yellow raisins
1	cup chickpeas, drained and rinsed
2	tsp turmeric
2	tsp pumpkin pie spice
1	tsp thyme
	Salt and fresh ground pepper to taste
1	5.9-oz box couscous, cooked according to package directions (no fat added)

1. In a large nonstick saucepot over medium-high heat, heat the oil. Add the vegetables, onion, and garlic and sauté for 5 minutes.

2. Reduce the heat to low, add remaining ingredients except the couscous, and cook for 10 minutes, stirring frequently.

3. Make a bed of prepared couscous on a platter. Top with vegetable mixture and serve.

Exchanges

4 Starch
1/2 Fruit
1 Monounsaturated Fat

Calories 396
   Calories from Fat . . 75
Total Fat . . . . 8 g
   Saturated Fat . . . . . . 2 g
Cholesterol . . . . 0 mg
Sodium . . . . 101 mg
Carbohydrate . . . . . . 70 g
   Dietary Fiber . . . . . 10 g
   Sugars . . . . 15 g
Protein . . . . 13 g

Tuna Penne

Serves 4   Serving size: 3–4 oz tuna, 1 cup pasta and vegetables
Preparation time: 15 minutes
Cooking time: 10 minutes

FROZEN FOODS: fish, peppers and onions

ALSO VISIT: shelves for vinegar, olives, penne pasta; produce for basil, parsley

4   4-oz frozen tuna fillets, defrosted in refrigerator overnight

1/2   of 1-lb bag frozen bell peppers and onions

2   Tbsp olive oil

1/4   cup red wine vinegar

2   Tbsp chopped fresh basil

2   Tbsp chopped fresh parsley

1/2   cup chopped black olives

Salt and fresh ground pepper to taste

4   cups cooked penne pasta

1. Defrost the peppers and onions.

2. Heat the oil in a large skillet over medium-high heat. Add the fish, onions, peppers, vinegar, basil, parsley, olives, salt, and pepper. Cook, covered, over medium-high heat for about 5 minutes. Remove tuna from skillet; keep warm.

3. Reduce liquid remaining in skillet over medium heat for 5 minutes. Serve tuna and sauce over penne pasta.

Exchanges
3 Starch
4 Lean Meat
1/2 Monounsaturated Fat

Calories 492
    Calories from Fat . 166
Total Fat . . . . 18 g
    Saturated Fat . . . . . 2 g
Cholesterol . . . . 44 mg
Sodium . . . . 287 mg
Carbohydrate . . . . . 46 g
    Dietary Fiber . . . . . 4 g
    Sugars . . . . 4 g
Protein . . . . 34 g

Caribbean Chicken Breasts

Serves 4   Serving size: 3–4 oz with sauce
Preparation time: 5 minutes
Cooking time: 15 minutes
Standing time: 5 hours or overnight

FROZEN FOODS: chicken, orange juice concentrate

ALSO VISIT: shelves for orange, spices, lime juice

> 2 Tbsp frozen orange juice concentrate
> 1 tsp grated orange peel
> 1 Tbsp olive oil
> 2 tsp lime juice
> 1 tsp ground ginger
> 2 tsp minced garlic
> 1/2 tsp oregano
> 1/2 tsp white pepper
>   Salt and fresh ground pepper to taste
> 4 4-oz portions frozen boneless, skinless chicken breasts

1. Combine all ingredients except the chicken in a large bowl. Add chicken to marinade. Refrigerate 5 hours or overnight.

2. Discard the marinade and grill or broil the chicken for 5–7 minutes per side, until juices run clear.

Exchanges
4 Very Lean Meat

Calories 148
  Calories from Fat . . 36
Total Fat . . . . 4 g
  Saturated Fat . . . . . . 1 g
Cholesterol . . . . 68 mg
Sodium . . . . 60 mg
Carbohydrate . . . . 1 g
  Dietary Fiber . . . . . . 0 g
  Sugars . . . . 1 g
Protein . . . . 25 g

Salmon Tortellini Salad

Serves 4   Serving size: 1 1/2 cups
Preparation time: 15 minutes
Cooking time: 10 minutes
Standing time: 1–2 hours

FROZEN FOODS: tortellini, peas

ALSO VISIT: shelves for artichokes, mustard, lemon juice, roasted red pepper, mayonnaise; seafood department for salmon; dairy case for sour cream; salad bar for green onion

  1   1-lb pkg frozen tortellini (vegetable- or cheese-filled works best)

  1   cup frozen peas, defrosted

1/2   cup fat-free sour cream

  1   14-oz can water-packed artichokes, chopped

  2   Tbsp chopped green onion

  2   tsp dried dill

  2   tsp Dijon mustard

  1   Tbsp lemon juice

1/4   tsp chopped fresh parsley

  1   roasted red pepper from jar, chopped

1/4   cup low-fat mayonnaise

  2   cloves garlic, minced

      Salt and fresh ground pepper to taste

  1   15.5-oz can salmon, drained, deboned, and flaked

1. Prepare tortellini according to directions. Cool.

2. Combine all ingredients except salmon and tortellini in a medium bowl.

3. Mix salmon and tortellini together in a large bowl. Add the mixture of other ingredients and toss together. Refrigerate for 1–2 hours before serving.

Exchanges
4 Starch
3 Lean Meat
1/2 Fat

Calories 528
  Calories from Fat . 134
Total Fat . . . . 15 g
  Saturated Fat . . . . . . 2 g
Cholesterol . . . . 97 mg
Sodium . . . . 1395 mg
Carbohydrate . . . . . . 59 g
  Dietary Fiber . . . . . . 4 g
  Sugars . . . . 12 g
Protein . . . . 39 g

Spinach Casserole Au Gratin

Serves 4   Serving size: 1 cup
Preparation time: 10 minutes
Cooking time: 1 hour

FROZEN FOODS: spinach

ALSO VISIT: shelves for artichoke hearts, broth; produce for onion, garlic; dairy case for sour cream, Parmesan cheese, eggs

1	14-oz can water-packed artichoke hearts, drained and finely chopped
1/4	cup low-fat, low-sodium chicken broth
1	10-oz pkg frozen chopped spinach, thawed and drained
2	Tbsp minced onion
1	Tbsp chopped garlic
1/2	tsp black pepper
1/2	cup fat-free sour cream
1/4	cup grated Parmesan cheese
2	eggs, beaten
	Butter-flavored nonstick cooking spray

1. Preheat oven to 350°F.

2. Combine all ingredients.

3. Spray a soufflé dish with butter-flavored nonstick cooking spray. Pour ingredients into dish. Bake for 1 hour, until golden brown and bubbly.

Exchanges
1/2 Carbohydrate
2 Vegetable
1 Saturated Fat

Calories 142
   Calories from Fat . . 47
Total Fat . . . . 5 g
   Saturated Fat . . . . . . 3 g
Cholesterol . . . . 116 mg
Sodium . . . . 483 mg
Carbohydrate . . . . . . 15 g
   Dietary Fiber . . . . . . 3 g
   Sugars . . . . 5 g
Protein . . . . 11 g

Orange Ginger Chicken

Serves 4   Serving size: 4 oz
Preparation time: 10 minutes
Cooking time: 15 minutes
Standing time: 4 hours

FROZEN FOODS: chicken, orange juice concentrate

ALSO VISIT: shelves for sherry, spices, honey

1/2	cup dry sherry
1/2	tsp white pepper
1/2	tsp ground ginger
2	cloves garlic, minced
1/4	tsp grated orange peel
3	Tbsp frozen orange juice concentrate
1/4	cup water
2	tsp honey
4	4-oz portions frozen boneless, skinless chicken breasts

1. In a large bowl, whisk together all the ingredients except the chicken.

2. Add the chicken breasts. Cover and marinate in the refrigerator for at least 4 hours or overnight.

3. Preheat the oven broiler. Discard the marinade and broil the chicken 4 inches away from the heat for about 5–7 minutes per side, until juices run clear.

Exchanges
4 Very Lean Meat

Calories 151
  Calories from Fat . . 26
Total Fat . . . . 3 g
  Saturated Fat . . . . . . 1 g
Cholesterol . . . . 68 mg
Sodium . . . . 61 mg
Carbohydrate . . . . 3 g
  Dietary Fiber . . . . . . 0 g
  Sugars . . . . 3 g
Protein . . . . 25 g

Roasted Game Hens with Savory Vegetable Stuffing

Serves 4   Serving size: 1/2 hen, 1/2 cup stuffing
Preparation time: 20 minutes
Cooking time: 45 minutes (add 20 minutes if rice is not already prepared)

FROZEN FOODS: Cornish hens

ALSO VISIT: shelves for jelly, mustard, spices, rice

Stuffing:
- 1 cup cooked white rice (can use leftover rice)
- 2 Tbsp minced garlic
- 1/2 tsp ground sage
- 2 tsp olive oil
- 1 pkg (1/2-lb) frozen mixed vegetables

Glaze:
- 1/2 cup no-added-sugar apricot jelly
- 1 Tbsp Dijon mustard
- Salt and fresh ground pepper to taste
- 2 14-oz frozen Cornish game hens, defrosted, washed, halved, and skinned (giblets removed)

1. Preheat oven to 350°F.

2. In a large bowl, mix together rice, garlic, sage, oil, and vegetables. Set aside.

3. In a small saucepan or in the microwave, heat the jelly until it melts. Add the mustard, salt, and pepper.

4. Spread the stuffing over the bottom of a nonstick casserole dish. Top with the Cornish game hen halves. Bake, uncovered, for 20 minutes. Brush the glaze over the hens. Continue to bake for another 15–20 minutes, brushing with glaze occasionally, until hens are cooked through and juices run clear.

Exchanges
2 Starch
4 Very Lean Meat

Calories	307
Calories from Fat	61
Total Fat	7 g
Saturated Fat	2 g
Cholesterol	117 mg
Sodium	163 mg
Carbohydrate	31 g
Dietary Fiber	2 g
Sugars	9 g
Protein	29 g

Seafood Fajitas

Serves 4   Serving size: 4 oz fish, 1 tortilla
Preparation time: 10 minutes
Cooking time: 10 minutes

FROZEN FOODS: fish, tortillas

ALSO VISIT: shelves for bean dip, salsa; dairy for sour cream

4 4-oz frozen Italian or lemon-pepper fish fillets

4 10-inch tortillas (frozen or refrigerated)

4 Tbsp fat-free bean dip

4 Tbsp fat-free sour cream

4 Tbsp salsa

4 Tbsp low-fat shredded cheddar cheese

1. Bake the fish according to the package directions.

2. Meanwhile, wrap the tortillas in foil. Place in the oven with the fish for 5 minutes. Remove the fish and tortillas from the oven.

3. Carefully spread each tortilla with the bean dip and sour cream. Flake fish and crumble on top. Add salsa and cheese. Fold over sides of tortilla and roll up end.

Exchanges

3 Starch
4 Very Lean Meat

Calories 377
　Calories from Fat . . 60
Total Fat . . . . 7 g
　Saturated Fat . . . . . . 2 g
Cholesterol . . . . 68 mg
Sodium . . . . 589 mg
Carbohydrate . . . . . . 46 g
　Dietary Fiber . . . . . . 3 g
　Sugars . . . . 3 g
Protein . . . . 31 g

Shrimp Ravioli Classico

Serves 4 Serving size: 1/2 cup ravioli, about 3 oz shrimp, 1/2 cup vegetables
Preparation time: 15 minutes
Cooking time: 20 minutes (includes boiling ravioli)

FROZEN FOODS: ravioli, peppers and onions, shrimp

ALSO VISIT: shelves for olive oil, Italian seasoning, marinara sauce, tomatoes; produce or salad bar for zucchini

2	cups frozen cheese ravioli
1	Tbsp olive oil
1	1-lb bag frozen peppers and onions
1/2	cup chopped zucchini
1	14-oz bag frozen salad shrimp, thawed
1	tsp Italian seasoning
1	cup jarred marinara sauce
1	14-oz can diced tomatoes, drained

1. Boil ravioli according to package directions. Drain and set aside.

2. In a large skillet over medium-high heat, heat the oil. Add the peppers and onions and zucchini. Sauté for 5 minutes.

3. Add the shrimp and sauté for 2 minutes. Add the Italian seasoning. Add the marinara sauce and diced tomatoes and bring to a boil.

4. Lower the heat and simmer for 5 minutes. Serve the mixture over the ravioli.

Exchanges

2 1/2 Starch
1 Vegetable
3 Very Lean Meat
1 Monounsaturated Fat

Calories 376
 Calories from Fat . . 92
Total Fat . . . . 10 g
 Saturated Fat . . . . . . 3 g
Cholesterol . . . . 153 mg
Sodium . . . . 687 mg
Carbohydrate . . . . . . 42 g
 Dietary Fiber . . . . . . 5 g
 Sugars . . . . 12 g
Protein . . . . 28 g

Italian Ravioli Soup

Serves 6   Serving size: about 1 cup
Preparation time: 20 minutes
Cooking time: 25 minutes

FROZEN FOODS: Italian vegetables, ravioli

ALSO VISIT: shelves for broth, Italian seasoning; salad bar or produce section for shredded cabbage, onion

2 cups frozen ravioli (meat or cheese)

1 Tbsp olive oil

1 medium onion, chopped

1 Tbsp Italian seasoning
    Salt and fresh ground pepper to taste

1 1-lb pkg frozen Italian vegetables

1 cup shredded cabbage

5 cups fat-free, reduced-sodium chicken broth

1. Boil the ravioli according to package directions. Drain and set aside.

2. In a large saucepot over medium-high heat, heat the olive oil. Add the onions and seasonings. Cook for 2–3 minutes.

3. Add the Italian vegetables and cabbage. Cook for another 3–4 minutes. Add broth and ravioli. Cook for another 15 minutes.

Exchanges
2 Starch
1 Very Lean Meat

Calories 192
    Calories from Fat . . 42
Total Fat . . . . 5 g
    Saturated Fat . . . . . . 2 g
Cholesterol . . . . 15 mg
Sodium . . . . 529 mg
Carbohydrate . . . . . . 27 g
    Dietary Fiber . . . . . . 3 g
    Sugars . . . . 5 g
Protein . . . . 10 g

Shrimp Rolls

Serves 6   Serving size: 3 oz with bun
Preparation time: 15 minutes

FROZEN FOODS: shrimp

ALSO VISIT: shelves for mayonnaise; bakery department for bread; salad bar for celery, green onions; produce for garlic

1	lb frozen cooked large shrimp, thawed
3	cloves garlic, minced
1/2	cup low-fat mayonnaise
1/2	cup sliced celery
1/2	cup minced green onions
1	Tbsp lemon juice
1	cup shredded romaine lettuce
6	whole-grain hamburger buns

1. Combine the cooked shrimp with all ingredients except the lettuce and buns.

2. On one side of each bun, scoop out some of the bread, leaving a hole with about 1 inch of shell surrounding it. Put some lettuce in the hole. Pile on the shrimp salad and top with remaining bread half.

Exchanges

2 Starch
2 Very Lean Meat

Calories 231
  Calories from Fat . . 38
Total Fat . . . . 4 g
  Saturated Fat . . . . . . 0 g
Cholesterol . . . . 126 mg
Sodium . . . . 584 mg
Carbohydrate . . . . . . 29 g
  Dietary Fiber . . . . . . 2 g
  Sugars . . . . 8 g
Protein . . . . 18 g

Shrimp, Tomato, and Pasta Salad

Serves 4   Serving size: 1 cup pasta, 3 oz shrimp
Preparation time: 20 minutes

FROZEN FOODS: shrimp

ALSO VISIT: shelves for sun-dried tomatoes, pasta; salad bar for tomatoes, spinach; produce for lemons, herbs

1	lb frozen cooked medium shrimp, thawed
12	sun-dried tomatoes, rehydrated and sliced
1	cup diced tomatoes
2	cups torn spinach
1/2	cup chopped Italian parsley
1/2	cup chopped fresh basil leaves
2	Tbsp olive oil
1/4	cup fresh lemon juice
	Fresh ground pepper and salt to taste
4	cups cooked bow tie noodles

Combine the shrimp with the remaining ingredients. Toss well and serve.

Exchanges

2 1/2 Starch
2 Vegetable
3 Very Lean Meat

Calories 380
   Calories from Fat . . 83
Total Fat . . . . 9 g
   Saturated Fat . . . . . . 2 g
Cholesterol . . . . 190 mg
Sodium . . . . 245 mg
Carbohydrate . . . . . . 45 g
   Dietary Fiber . . . . . . 5 g
   Sugars . . . . 9 g
Protein . . . . 29 g

Shrimp with Country Mustard Sauce

Serves 6   Serving size: 3 oz
Preparation time: 35 minutes

FROZEN FOODS: shrimp

ALSO VISIT: shelves for oil, broth, mustard, evaporated skim milk, flour, wine; produce for garlic, shallots

2	tsp olive oil
2	shallots, minced
2	cloves garlic, minced
2	Tbsp unbleached flour
1/4	cup white wine
1/4	cup low-fat, low-sodium chicken broth
1	12-oz can evaporated fat-free milk
2	Tbsp coarse Dijon mustard
	Salt and fresh ground pepper to taste
1	lb frozen large cooked shrimp, thawed

Garnish: 2 Tbsp minced parsley

1. In a large skillet over medium-high heat, heat the oil. Add the shallots and garlic and sauté for 3 minutes. Add the flour and sauté for 1 minute.

2. Add the broth and wine and cook for 2–3 minutes over medium heat. Add the milk and lower the heat to medium-low. Cook until thickened, about 3–4 minutes.

3. Add the mustard, salt, and pepper and cook 1 minute. Add the shrimp and cook 1 minute. Garnish with minced parsley.

Exchanges

1/2 Starch
1/2 Fat Free Milk
2 Very Lean Meat

Calories	151
Calories from Fat	23
Total Fat	3 g
Saturated Fat	0 g
Cholesterol	126 mg
Sodium	309 mg
Carbohydrate	11 g
Dietary Fiber	0 g
Sugars	7 g
Protein	19 g

Chinese Ginger Shrimp

Serves 6   Serving size: 3–4 oz, 1/2 cup rice
Preparation time: 20 minutes

FROZEN FOODS: shrimp

ALSO VISIT: shelves for oil, broth, soy sauce, vinegar, cornstarch, spices; produce for ginger, garlic, green onions

1 1/2	lb frozen peeled, cooked jumbo shrimp
1	tsp corn oil
2	green onions, minced
2	tsp minced ginger root
2	cloves garlic, minced
3/4	cup low-sodium, low-fat chicken broth
3	Tbsp lite soy sauce
2	Tbsp apple cider vinegar
2	tsp rice vinegar
1/4	tsp chili powder
1	Tbsp cornstarch or arrowroot
2	Tbsp water
3	cups cooked brown rice

1. In a large skillet, over medium-high heat, heat the oil. Add the green onions, ginger, and garlic. Stir-fry for 30 seconds.

2. Add the broth, soy sauce, cider vinegar, rice vinegar, and chili powder. Bring to a boil. Lower the heat. Add the shrimp and cook for 3–4 minutes, turning shrimp once.

3. Mix the cornstarch or arrowroot with the water. Add to the skillet and cook until thickened. Serve the shrimp over the rice.

Exchanges
1 1/2 Starch
3 Very Lean Meat

Calories	226
Calories from Fat	. . 24
Total Fat	3 g
Saturated Fat	0 g
Cholesterol	189 mg
Sodium	586 mg
Carbohydrate	26 g
Dietary Fiber	2 g
Sugars	2 g
Protein	24 g

Vegetarian Tri-Color Tortellini Salad

Serves 4   Serving size: 1 cup pasta, about 1 cup vegetables
Preparation time: 15 minutes
Standing time: several hours

FROZEN FOODS: tortellini, corn, peas

ALSO VISIT: salad bar for red bell pepper, tomatoes; shelves for artichoke hearts, vinegar, spices; produce for parsley, chives

4 cups frozen tortellini (preferably stuffed with vegetables rather than cheese), cooked according to package directions

1 cup diced red bell pepper

1 cup chopped tomatoes

1/2 cup chopped water-packed artichoke hearts, drained

1/2 cup frozen corn, thawed

1/2 cup frozen peas, thawed

2 Tbsp minced parsley

Dressing:
1/2 cup balsamic vinegar

2 Tbsp olive oil

2 tsp minced chives

Fresh ground pepper and salt to taste

1. Combine the salad ingredients together in a large salad bowl.

2. Whisk together the dressing ingredients and pour over the salad. Chill for several hours before serving.

Exchanges

4 Starch
2 Monounsaturated Fat

Calories 410
    Calories from Fat . 128
Total Fat . . . . 14 g
    Saturated Fat . . . . . . 4 g
Cholesterol . . . . 35 mg
Sodium . . . . 424 mg
Carbohydrate . . . . . . 57 g
    Dietary Fiber . . . . . . 4 g
    Sugars . . . . 11 g
Protein . . . . 16 g

Shrimp, Corn, and Pepper Sauté

Serves 4   Serving size: 3–4 oz shrimp, 2/3 cup vegetables
Preparation time: 15 minutes
Cooking time: 15 minutes

FROZEN FOODS: shrimp, corn

ALSO VISIT: salad bar for bell peppers, cherry tomatoes; shelves for lemon juice; produce for fresh basil

1	Tbsp canola oil
1/2	cup chopped onion
1	cup frozen corn
1/2	cup diced red bell pepper
1/2	cup diced green bell pepper
1/2	cup halved cherry tomatoes
2	Tbsp fresh lemon juice
1	lb frozen cooked shrimp, thawed
2	Tbsp minced fresh basil
	Fresh black pepper and salt to taste

1. In a large skillet over medium heat, heat the oil. Add the onion and sauté for 5 minutes. Add the corn and peppers and sauté for 5 minutes.

2. Add the cherry tomatoes and lemon juice. Cover, reduce heat to low, and cook for 3 minutes.

3. Add the shrimp, basil, black pepper, and salt and cook 1 more minute.

Exchanges
1/2 Starch
1 Vegetable
3 Very Lean Meat

Calories 185
  Calories from Fat . . 45
Total Fat . . . . 5 g
  Saturated Fat . . . . . . 0 g
Cholesterol . . . . 190 mg
Sodium . . . . 224 mg
Carbohydrate . . . . . . 14 g
  Dietary Fiber . . . . . . 2 g
  Sugars . . . . 3 g
Protein . . . . 22 g

Recipes Using Shelf-Stable Foods

TODAY THERE IS MORE THAN BOXED MACARONI and cheese available for dinner. This chapter uses four main boxed or canned products I would recommend every cook have on hand for quick dinners: pasta, rice, couscous, and beans. These four can provide the basis for many healthy meals. These products have a shelf life of up to a year, making them ideal foods to store in your pantry.

In the pasta recipes, I like to use different shapes to add interest and fun to the dishes. If you enjoy whole-wheat pasta, feel free to use that instead. Here are a few of my favorite pasta tips.

- Serve pasta at room temperature rather than steaming hot. Pasta is tastier served a bit cooler.

- When you cook pasta, make sure your pot is at a full rolling boil. Otherwise your pasta will not cook properly.

- You do not need to rinse pasta before adding sauce. You are rinsing off starch that helps the sauce adhere.

- Cook your pasta "al dente," meaning "to the tooth." Most people like it best slightly chewy.

- Use chunky sauces with shaped pastas and smoother sauces with thin pastas.

- I don't add oil to my pasta as it cooks. Smaller-shaped pasta has less of a tendency to stick together. Gently separate the strands of pasta and then coat with sauce to keep them from sticking together.

Couscous is a staple of Middle Eastern cuisine. It is the granular form of semolina (wheat pasta). Sometimes you will see it labeled as Moroccan pasta, as it is used in Morocco the same way pasta is used here. Now, couscous is available with interesting flavors. Since couscous is basically a blank canvas with not much taste on its own, the new flavored versions are quite delicious. Be sure to buy the precooked, 5-minute-style couscous.

You will need to rehydrate it for these recipes. (The cooking time listed includes the rehydration time.)

I use mainly white rice here because it cooks more quickly, but feel free to use brown rice if you have time. The best way to test rice for doneness is simply to taste it. If the liquid is all absorbed and the rice is tender, it is done. Be sure to have a lid that fits. Rice needs a fully enclosed vessel, so steam can build and cause the grains of rice to properly swell. And avoid at all costs the temptation to play chef and stir while the rice cooks. If you stir rice while it cooks, you release the starch in the grain, which causes the rice to become sticky and gummy.

I like to use canned beans, again to save time. You can certainly soak and cook your own dried beans if you like. Beans, when combined with rice or another grain, are a great alternative to meat. Beans provide an impressive amount of fiber, too, anywhere from 4–10 grams of fiber per cup.

*R*ecipes

Recipes Using Shelf-Stable Foods   **141**

Couscous Vegetable Pilaf with Roasted Chicken

Serves 4   **Serving size: 1/2 cup couscous, 4 oz chicken, 1/2 cup vegetables**
Preparation time: 15 minutes
Cooking time: 10 minutes

SHELF-STABLE FOODS: broth, couscous, spices

ALSO VISIT: salad bar for zucchini, carrots, onion; deli for chicken; produce for parsley

2	tsp olive oil
1/4	cup minced onion
3	cloves garlic, minced
1	medium zucchini, diced, peel on
1	medium carrot, diced
1/2	tsp Italian seasoning
1/4	tsp fresh ground black pepper
2	cups low-fat, low-sodium chicken broth
1	cup couscous
1	lb cooked diced roasted chicken

Garnish: 2 Tbsp minced parsley

1. In a large skillet over medium-high heat, heat the oil. Add the onion and garlic and sauté for 3 minutes.

2. Add the zucchini and carrots, reduce the heat to medium, and sauté for 5 minutes. Add the Italian seasoning, salt, pepper, and broth; bring to a boil.

3. Add the couscous. Remove from heat, cover, and let the mixture stand for 5–7 minutes. Add the chicken and return to the heat to heat through. Garnish with minced parsley.

Exchanges
2 1/2 Starch
1 Vegetable
4 Lean Meat

Calories 429
    Calories from Fat . 100
Total Fat . . . . 11 g
    Saturated Fat . . . . . . 3 g
Cholesterol . . . . 100 mg
Sodium . . . . 1186 mg
Carbohydrate . . . . . . 39 g
    Dietary Fiber . . . . . . 4 g
    Sugars . . . . 5 g
Protein . . . . 41 g

Italian Penne and Shrimp Salad

Serves 4   Serving size: 1/2 cup penne, 3 oz shrimp
Preparation time: 20 minutes
**Cooking time: 8–9 minutes to cook penne (or as directed on
       package)**

SHELF-STABLE FOODS: penne noodles, artichoke hearts, roasted red
bell peppers, capers, olives, salad dressing

ALSO VISIT: frozen foods or seafood department for shrimp; produce for
parsley, basil

- 2 cups cooked penne noodles
- 1 14-oz can artichoke hearts, drained and halved
- 2 roasted red bell peppers from jar, diced
- 2 tsp capers
- 1/2 cup pitted Kalamata olives
- 12 oz cooked medium shrimp, peeled and deveined
- 2 Tbsp minced fresh Italian parsley
- 2 Tbsp minced fresh basil
- 3/4 cup fat-free Italian salad dressing
- Salt and fresh ground pepper to taste

Combine all ingredients and chill for
1 hour in the refrigerator before serving.

Exchanges
2 Starch
3 Very Lean Meat

Calories 250
  Calories from Fat . . 32
Total Fat . . . . 4 g
  Saturated Fat . . . . . . 0 g
Cholesterol . . . . 165 mg
Sodium . . . . 1052 mg
Carbohydrate . . . . . . 31 g
  Dietary Fiber . . . . . . 3 g
  Sugars . . . . 8 g
Protein . . . . 23 g

Couscous Marinara

Serves 4 Serving size: 1/2 cup couscous, 4 oz shrimp, 1/2 cup vegetables

Preparation time: 15 minutes Cooking time: 20 minutes

SHELF-STABLE FOODS: couscous, broth, canned tomatoes, spices, tomato paste, wine

ALSO VISIT: salad bar for onion, green pepper, mushrooms; frozen foods for shrimp

1 cup couscous	
2 tsp olive oil	**Exchanges**
1 cup diced onion	3 Starch
2 cloves garlic, minced	1 Vegetable
1 cup diced green pepper	3 Very Lean Meat
3 cups sliced mushrooms	
1 15-oz can Italian-style diced tomatoes, with juices	**Calories** 373
	Calories from Fat . . 39
	Total Fat . . . . 4 g
2 Tbsp tomato paste	Saturated Fat . . . . . . 1 g
2 Tbsp white wine	**Cholesterol** . . . . 220 mg
	Sodium . . . . 941 mg
1/4 tsp crushed red pepper	**Carbohydrate** . . . . . . 48 g
1/4 tsp fresh ground black pepper	Dietary Fiber . . . . . . 5 g
	Sugars . . . . 9 g
1 lb cooked medium shrimp	**Protein** . . . . 34 g

1. Place the couscous in a heatproof bowl. Add the broth and cover. Set aside while you prepare the marinara mixture.

2. In a skillet over medium-high heat, heat the oil. Add the onion and garlic and sauté for 3 minutes. Add the green pepper and mushrooms and sauté for 5 minutes until mushrooms have browned.

3. Add the canned tomatoes, tomato paste, white wine, crushed red pepper, black pepper, and salt. Simmer for 5 minutes. Add the shrimp and cook for 1 minute.

4. Mound the couscous on a serving platter. Serve the shrimp marinara over the couscous.

Vegetarian Couscous and Chickpea Pilaf

Serves 4   Serving size: 1/2 cup couscous, 1/2 cup chickpeas, 1/2 cup vegetables
Preparation time: 15 minutes   Cooking time: 20 minutes

SHELF-STABLE FOODS: chickpeas, broth, couscous, hot sauce, spices

ALSO VISIT: salad bar for red onion, carrot; produce for garlic; frozen foods for spinach (or produce for fresh spinach)

2   tsp olive oil

1/2 cup diced red onion

1   clove garlic, minced

1   large carrot, diced

2   medium tomatoes, diced

1   cup chopped fresh spinach or frozen spinach, thawed and well drained (squeeze out all the water)

2   tsp lemon juice

1/4 tsp salt

1/4 tsp fresh ground black pepper

1/2 tsp dried thyme

2   cups canned chickpeas, rinsed and drained

2   cups low-fat, low-sodium vegetable broth

1   cup couscous

1/8 tsp hot sauce

Exchanges

4 Starch
1 Vegetable
1/2 Monounsaturated Fat

Calories 359
  Calories from Fat . . 45
Total Fat . . . . 5 g
  Saturated Fat . . . . . . 1 g
Cholesterol . . . . 0 mg
Sodium . . . . 600 mg
Carbohydrate . . . . . . 64 g
  Dietary Fiber . . . . . 10 g
  Sugars . . . . 10 g
Protein . . . . 16 g

1. In a skillet over medium-high heat, heat oil. Add onion and garlic and sauté 3 minutes. Add carrots and sauté 3–5 minutes, stirring occasionally. Add tomatoes and spinach and cook 3 minutes, until the spinach is wilted but not overcooked.

2. Add lemon juice, salt, pepper, and thyme. Stir to coat. Add chickpeas and broth and bring to a boil. Add couscous. Cover and remove from heat for 5–7 minutes until couscous absorbs the broth; then add hot sauce.

Couscous Paella

**Serves 4   Serving size: 1/2 cup couscous, 1/2 cup vegetables,
1 oz shrimp, 1 oz chicken, 1 oz clams**
Preparation time: 15 minutes   Cooking time: 17 minutes

SHELF-STABLE FOODS: broth, saffron, spices, couscous, clams

ALSO VISIT: salad bar for red onion, bell peppers, tomatoes; frozen foods
for peas, shrimp; deli or meat department for chicken; produce for parsley,
garlic

2 tsp olive oil	
1/2 cup diced red onion	**Exchanges**
3 cloves garlic, minced	2 1/2 Starch
1/2 cup diced green bell pepper	2 Vegetable 3 Very Lean Meat
1 cup diced red bell pepper	
1/2 cup frozen peas	**Calories** . . . . 345 Calories from Fat . . 42
1 1/2 cups low-sodium, low-fat chicken broth	**Total Fat** . . . . 5 g Saturated Fat . . . . . . 1 g
1/4 tsp saffron threads	**Cholesterol** . . . . 93 mg
1/4 tsp salt	**Sodium** . . . . 513 mg **Carbohydrate** . . . . . . 46 g
1/2 tsp fresh ground black pepper	**Dietary Fiber** . . . . . . 5 g Sugars . . . . 7 g **Protein** . . . . 29 g
1/4 lb cooked medium shrimp	

1/4 lb diced cooked boneless skinless chicken breast

1 6.5-oz can chopped clams, drained

1 cup couscous

1 medium tomato, diced

Garnish: 2 Tbsp minced parsley

1. In a large skillet over medium-high heat, heat oil. Add onion and garlic
and sauté 2–3 minutes. Add peppers and sauté 3–5 minutes, stirring
often.

2. Add peas, broth, saffron, salt, and pepper and bring to boil. Add shrimp,
chicken, and clams and heat 1 minute. Stir in couscous and remove from
heat. Add tomato, cover, and let stand 5–7 minutes. Fluff with fork and
garnish with parsley.

Cool Couscous and Roasted Red Pepper Dinner Salad

Serves 4   Serving size: 2 cups
Preparation time: 20 minutes   Cooking time: 10 minutes
Standing time: 1 hour

SHELF-STABLE FOODS: couscous, broth, jarred roasted red peppers, artichoke hearts, sun-dried tomatoes, balsamic vinegar, spices

ALSO VISIT: salad bar for carrots, green onions; deli for turkey

1 cup	couscous
1 1/2 cups	low-fat, low-sodium chicken broth, boiling
1 cup	thinly sliced jarred roasted red pepper
1/4 cup	sliced green onions
6	artichoke hearts, canned in water, drained and quartered
1/2 cup	diced sun-dried tomato (rehydrated or packed in oil) or fresh tomato
1/2 cup	thinly sliced carrots
1 lb	diced cooked turkey breast
1 Tbsp	olive oil
2 Tbsp	balsamic vinegar
1 Tbsp	lemon juice
1/2 tsp	dried oregano
1/2 tsp	dried basil
1/4 tsp	dried thyme
1/4 tsp	fresh ground black pepper

Exchanges

3 Starch
4 Very Lean Meat

Calories	381
Calories from Fat	69
Total Fat	8 g
Saturated Fat	2 g
Cholesterol	52 mg
Sodium	1464 mg
Carbohydrate	47 g
Dietary Fiber	5 g
Sugars	8 g
Protein	34 g

1. Place couscous in a heatproof bowl. Pour boiling chicken broth over couscous and cover. Let stand 5–10 minutes until couscous has absorbed the broth.

2. Add pepper, onions, artichoke hearts, tomatoes, carrots, and turkey to couscous. Toss well. In a separate bowl, whisk together remaining ingredients. Pour dressing over couscous mixture and refrigerate for 1 hour.

Pesto Couscous with Garden Vegetables and Shrimp

Serves 4   Serving size: 1/2 cup couscous, 1 cup vegetables, 4 oz shrimp

Preparation time: 15 minutes   Cooking time: 25 minutes

SHELF-STABLE FOODS: broth, spices, pesto, couscous

ALSO VISIT: salad bar for zucchini, yellow squash, carrots; produce (or frozen foods) for green beans; frozen foods for shrimp

2	tsp olive oil
1	small onion, diced
2	cloves garlic, minced
1	cup sliced zucchini
1	cup sliced yellow squash
1	cup thinly sliced carrots
1	cup trimmed green beans, cut into 2-inch pieces
1	cup couscous
1 1/2	cups low-fat, low-sodium chicken broth
1/4	tsp salt
1/4	tsp fresh ground black pepper
1/4	tsp Italian dry seasoning
2	Tbsp prepared pesto
1	lb cooked, shelled and deveined medium shrimp

Exchanges

2 1/2 Starch
2 Vegetable
3 Very Lean Meat

Calories 367
  Calories from Fat . . 55
Total Fat . . . . 6 g
  Saturated Fat . . . . . . 1 g
Cholesterol . . . . 220 mg
Sodium . . . . 680 mg
Carbohydrate . . . . . . 44 g
  Dietary Fiber . . . . . . 6 g
  Sugars . . . . 7 g
Protein . . . . 33 g

1. In a skillet over medium heat, heat oil. Add onion and garlic and sauté 2–3 minutes. Add zucchini, yellow squash, carrots, and green beans. Sauté 5–7 minutes until vegetables are tender yet crisp.

2. Add couscous and sauté 1 minute. Add broth, salt, pepper, and Italian seasoning and bring to a boil. Cover. Remove skillet from heat and keep covered for 5–10 minutes until couscous has absorbed the broth. Add pesto and shrimp to the skillet, return to medium heat, and heat 1 minute.

Asian-Style Couscous with Chicken and Vegetables

Serves 4   Serving size: 1/2 cup couscous, 1 cup vegetables, 3 oz chicken
Preparation time: 20 minutes
Cooking time: 27 minutes
Standing time: at least 30 minutes

SHELF-STABLE FOODS: sesame oil, couscous, broth, soy sauce, rice vinegar, sugar, hoisin sauce, sesame seeds

ALSO VISIT: salad bar for green onions, mushrooms (may need to go to produce for shiitake), carrot, zucchini, broccoli; produce for green beans (or use frozen and thawed), garlic, shallot, ginger root; meat department for chicken

1	Tbsp sesame oil, divided
1/4	cup minced green onion
2	tsp minced fresh ginger root
1	clove garlic, minced
1	small shallot, minced
1	lb cubed boneless, skinless chicken breasts
1/2	cup sliced shiitake mushrooms, stems removed, or sliced button mushrooms
1	cup thinly sliced or shredded carrot
1	cup thinly sliced zucchini
1	cup broccoli florets
1	cup trimmed green beans, cut into 2-inch lengths
1	cup couscous
1 1/2	cups low-fat, low-sodium chicken broth
1/4	cup lite soy sauce
1	Tbsp rice vinegar
2	tsp sugar
1	tsp hoisin sauce

Garnish: 2 Tbsp toasted sesame seeds; 2 Tbsp minced green onions

1. In a large wok or heavy skillet over medium-high heat, heat 1 tsp of the sesame oil. Add the green onion, ginger, garlic, and shallot and stir-fry for 3–4 minutes until aromatic. Add the chicken and stir-fry until it is no longer pink inside, about 5–7 minutes. Remove chicken and set aside.

2. Add 1/2 tsp of oil to the wok and heat over medium-high. Add the mushrooms and stir-fry until they are golden, about 3–4 minutes. Move mushrooms to the side of the wok, add 1/2 tsp of oil, heat, and add the carrots, zucchini, broccoli, and green beans. Cook for 5–8 minutes or until the vegetables are crisp-tender. Add the couscous and stir-fry for 1 minute.

3. Add the broth, bring to a boil, cover, and remove from the heat. Let couscous stand covered for 5–8 minutes until it has absorbed the broth. Return chicken to wok.

4. Combine the soy sauce, rice vinegar, sugar, remaining 1 tsp sesame oil, and hoisin sauce in a measuring cup. Mix well. Stir into the couscous mixture. Remove the couscous from the wok and place in a serving bowl. Chill for at least 30 minutes. Garnish each serving with toasted sesame seeds and minced green onions.

Exchanges

2 1/2 Starch
2 Vegetable
3 Lean Meat

Calories 415
   Calories from Fat . . 82
Total Fat . . . . 9 g
   Saturated Fat . . . . . . 2 g
Cholesterol . . . . 68 mg
Sodium . . . . 948 mg
Carbohydrate . . . . . . 48 g
   Dietary Fiber . . . . . . 6 g
   Sugars . . . . 9 g
Protein . . . . 35 g

Island Couscous with Chicken and Vegetables

Note: This dish is hot!

Serves 4   Serving size: 1/2 cup couscous, 3/4 cup vegetables, 3 oz chicken

Preparation time: 20 minutes

Cooking time: 25 minutes

SHELF-STABLE FOODS: sesame oil, jerk seasoning, couscous, broth, spices, mango chutney, lime juice

ALSO VISIT: salad bar for onions, carrots, tomatoes; produce for ginger root, kale (or use frozen kale); frozen foods for peas

2	tsp sesame oil
1	cup diced onions
2	tsp minced ginger root
1	lb boneless, skinless chicken tenders (cubed) or cubed chicken breast
2	tsp jerk seasoning
1	tsp lime juice
1	tsp dried thyme
1 1/2	cups thinly sliced carrots
1	cup frozen peas, thawed
1/2	cup finely chopped kale
1	cup couscous
1 1/2	cups low-fat, low-sodium chicken broth
1/2	tsp paprika
1	cup chopped, seeded tomatoes

Garnish: 1/4 cup mango chutney (optional)

1. In a heavy skillet over medium-high heat, heat the oil. Add the onions and ginger and sauté for 2–4 minutes. Add the chicken and sauté for 5 minutes, or until chicken is cooked and no pink remains.

2. Add the jerk seasoning, lime juice, and thyme. Toss to coat the chicken and sauté for 1 minute.

3. Add the carrots, peas, and kale and sauté for 3–4 minutes. Add the couscous and sauté for 1 minute.

4. Add the broth and paprika and bring to a boil. Remove the skillet from the heat and cover. Let stand for 5–8 minutes until the couscous has absorbed the broth.

5. Toss in the chopped tomatoes and garnish with mango chutney if desired.

Exchanges
3 Starch
1 Vegetable
3 Very Lean Meat
1/2 Fat

Calories 402
   Calories from Fat . . 52
Total Fat . . . . 6 g
   Saturated Fat . . . . . . 1 g
Cholesterol . . . . 68 mg
Sodium . . . . 491 mg
Carbohydrate . . . . . . 51 g
   Dietary Fiber . . . . . . 7 g
   Sugars . . . . 11 g
Protein . . . . 35 g

Refried Bean Pizzas

Serves 4 Serving size: 1/2 cup beans, 1 tortilla, 2 Tbsp salsa
Preparation time: 15 minutes Cooking time: 23 minutes

SHELF-STABLE FOODS: canned beans, spices, green chilies, olives, salsa

ALSO VISIT: salad bar for onions; produce for garlic, cilantro; refrigerated section for cheese, tortillas

- 2 tsp olive oil
- 1 small onion, minced
- 2 cloves garlic, minced
- 1 can (15 1/2 oz) black beans or pinto beans, rinsed, drained, and coarsely mashed with a potato masher
- 2 tsp chili powder
- 1/2 tsp cumin
- 1/4 tsp oregano
- 2 tsp minced cilantro
- Nonstick cooking spray
- 4 8-inch whole-wheat tortillas
- 1 cup low-fat shredded cheddar or Monterey Jack cheese
- 1 4.5-oz can diced green chilies
- 1 4.5-oz can sliced black olives
- 1/2 cup salsa

Exchanges

3 Starch
1 Vegetable
1 Very Lean Meat
2 Monounsaturated Fat

Calories 382
  Calories from Fat . 120
Total Fat . . . . 13 g
  Saturated Fat . . . . . . 3 g
Cholesterol . . . . 6 mg
Sodium . . . . 952 mg
Carbohydrate . . . . . . 49 g
  Dietary Fiber . . . . . 10 g
  Sugars . . . . 5 g
Protein . . . . 18 g

1. Preheat oven to 400°F. In a heavy skillet over medium-high heat, heat oil. Add onion and garlic and sauté 3 minutes. Add beans, chili powder, cumin, and oregano and cook over medium-high heat 5 minutes.

2. Raise heat to high and mash the beans again, but don't mash them completely. Cook over high heat until beans are slightly dry, about 5 minutes. Add cilantro.

3. Place 4 tortillas on a nonstick baking sheet. Spread bean mixture evenly over the tortillas. Top with cheese, chilies, and olives. Bake for 7–9 minutes. Serve with salsa.

Italian Tuna and White Bean Salad

Serves 4   Serving size: 1/2 cup beans, 1 cup vegetables, 1.5 oz tuna
Preparation time: 15 minutes
Standing time: 1 hour

SHELF-STABLE FOODS: canned beans, artichoke hearts, roasted red pepper, sun-dried tomatoes, balsamic vinegar, spices, tuna (or use from salad bar if available)

ALSO VISIT: frozen foods for green beans (or use fresh from produce section)

1   15.5-oz can cannellini or navy beans, drained and rinsed

1   cup sliced, water-packed artichoke hearts

1   cup sliced jarred roasted red pepper

1   cup frozen green beans, thawed, or fresh cooked green beans, trimmed

1   cup sliced sun-dried tomatoes (rehydrated, drained, and sliced)

1   6-oz can white-meat tuna, drained and flaked

2   Tbsp olive oil

3   Tbsp balsamic vinegar

2   tsp lemon juice

1/4   tsp dried oregano

1/2   tsp dried basil

1/4   tsp paprika

1/4   tsp salt

Fresh ground black pepper to taste

Combine all ingredients and chill in a serving bowl for 1 hour.

Exchanges
1 1/2 Starch
2 Vegetable
2 Lean Meat

Calories 276
   Calories from Fat . . 73
Total Fat . . . . 8 g
   Saturated Fat . . . . . . 2 g
Cholesterol . . . . 12 mg
Sodium . . . . 730 mg
Carbohydrate . . . . . . 34 g
   Dietary Fiber . . . . . . 8 g
   Sugars . . . . 9 g
Protein . . . . 20 g

Vegetarian Cassoulet

Serves 4   Serving size: 1 cup beans, 1 cup vegetables
Preparation time: 15 minutes
Cooking time: 22 minutes

SHELF-STABLE FOODS: canned beans, tomato sauce, brown sugar, molasses, spices

ALSO VISIT: salad bar for onion, carrots, celery; produce for garlic

- 2 tsp olive oil
- 1 medium onion, chopped
- 2 cups diced carrots
- 2 cups diced celery
- 2 cloves garlic, minced
- 2 15.5-oz cans great northern beans or navy beans, drained and rinsed
- 1 8-oz can tomato sauce
- 2 Tbsp brown sugar
- 1 Tbsp dark molasses
- 1/2 tsp allspice
- 1/4 tsp salt
- Fresh ground black pepper to taste

1. In a large skillet, over medium-high heat, heat the oil. Add the onion and sauté for 2 minutes. Add the carrots, celery, and garlic and sauté for 5 minutes, stirring occasionally.

2. Add the remaining ingredients. Reduce the heat to low and let simmer for 10–15 minutes.

Exchanges
3 1/2 Starch
2 Vegetable

Calories 339
  Calories from Fat . . 31
Total Fat . . . . 3 g
  Saturated Fat . . . . . . 1 g
Cholesterol . . . . 0 mg
Sodium . . . . 893 mg
Carbohydrate . . . . . . 65 g
  Dietary Fiber . . . . . 14 g
  Sugars . . . . 22 g
Protein . . . . 15 g

The Easiest Lentil Chili

Serves 4   Serving size: 1 1/2 cups
Preparation time: 15 minutes
Cooking time: 35 minutes

SHELF-STABLE FOODS: spices, canned tomatoes, broth, canned lentils, canned black beans

ALSO VISIT: salad bar for onion, carrots

2	tsp olive oil
1	medium onion, chopped
3	cloves garlic, minced
1/2	cup diced carrots
3	Tbsp medium-hot chili powder
1	tsp cumin
1	tsp dried oregano
1/4	tsp salt
1/4	tsp fresh ground black pepper
1	28-oz can plum tomatoes, coarsely chopped, in juice
1	14-oz can fat-free, reduced-sodium chicken or vegetable broth
1	cup canned lentils, rinsed and drained
1	cup black beans, rinsed and drained

1. In a saucepan over medium-high heat, heat the oil. Add the onion and garlic and sauté for 3 minutes. Add the carrots and sauté for 3 minutes more.

2. Add the chili powder, cumin, oregano, salt, and pepper and sauté for 1 minute. Add the tomatoes and broth and bring to a boil. Lower the heat and simmer for 15–20 minutes.

3. Add the lentils and black beans and simmer for 5 minutes.

Exchanges

2 Starch
1 Vegetable
1/2 Monounsaturated Fat

Calories 206
   Calories from Fat . . 35
Total Fat . . . . 4 g
   Saturated Fat . . . . . . 1 g
Cholesterol . . . . 0 mg
Sodium . . . . 860 mg
Carbohydrate . . . . . . 35 g
   Dietary Fiber . . . . . 12 g
   Sugars . . . . 12 g
Protein . . . . 12 g

Warm Turkey and White Bean Salad

Serves 4   Serving size: 1 3/4 cups
Preparation time: 10 minutes   Cooking time: 10 minutes

SHELF-STABLE FOODS: jarred roasted red peppers, canned beans, vinegar, pesto, walnuts

ALSO VISIT: deli for turkey; salad bar for mushrooms, green onion, lettuce; frozen foods for green beans; produce for garlic

- 1 Tbsp olive oil
- 2 cloves garlic, crushed (used to flavor pan)
- 1 cup sliced mushrooms
- 1/2 lb cooked turkey breast, cubed
- 1 cup sliced roasted red peppers from jar
- 1/2 cup sliced green onions
- 1 cup frozen cut green beans, thawed
- 1 15.5-oz can cannellini or navy beans, drained and rinsed
- 2 Tbsp red wine vinegar
- 2 Tbsp prepared pesto
- 1 small head romaine lettuce, torn into small pieces

Garnish: 1 Tbsp toasted chopped walnuts (optional)

1. In a skillet over medium-high heat, heat oil. Add crushed garlic and sauté 1 minute. Remove the garlic from the skillet and discard.

2. Add mushrooms and sauté 2–3 minutes. Add turkey and sauté 2 minutes. Add peppers, onions, and beans and cook 2 minutes. Add vinegar and pesto and heat thoroughly. Serve salad over lettuce. Garnish with walnuts if desired.

Exchanges

1 1/2 Starch
1 Vegetable
2 Lean Meat

Calories 256
  Calories from Fat . . 71
Total Fat . . . . 8 g
  Saturated Fat . . . . . . 2 g
Cholesterol . . . . 26 mg
Sodium . . . . 865 mg
Carbohydrate . . . . . . 28 g
  Dietary Fiber . . . . . . 8 g
  Sugars . . . . 6 g
Protein . . . . 21 g

Ginger Black Beans and Pasta

Serves 4   Serving size: 1/2 cup beans, 1/2 cup vegetables, 1/2 cup pasta

Preparation time: 10 minutes

Cooking time: 7 minutes (add 5–6 minutes for cooking angel hair pasta if not cooked before starting recipe)

SHELF-STABLE FOODS: sesame oil, black beans, angel hair pasta, spices

ALSO VISIT: salad bar for green onions, yellow and red bell peppers; produce for ginger root

- 2 tsp sesame oil
- 2 cloves garlic, minced
- 2 green onions, minced
- 1 Tbsp minced ginger root
- 2 cups diced combination yellow and red bell peppers
- 2 cups black beans, drained and rinsed
- Pinch cinnamon
- 2 cups cooked angel hair pasta

1. In a skillet or wok over medium-high heat, heat the oil. Add the garlic, green onions, and ginger and stir-fry for 1 minute. Add the peppers and sauté for 5 minutes.

2. Add the black beans and cinnamon. Simmer over low heat for 1 minute.

3. Serve the beans over angel hair pasta.

Exchanges

3 Starch
1 Vegetable

Calories 258
  Calories from Fat . . 30
Total Fat . . . . 3 g
  Saturated Fat . . . . . . 1 g
Cholesterol . . . . 0 mg
Sodium . . . . 158 mg
Carbohydrate . . . . . . 48 g
  Dietary Fiber . . . . . 10 g
  Sugars . . . . 5 g
Protein . . . . 12 g

15-Minute Chili

Serves 4   Serving size: 1 cup
Preparation time: 10 minutes
Cooking time: 15 minutes

SHELF-STABLE FOODS: canned beans, broth, canned tomatoes, tomato paste, spices

ALSO VISIT: meat department for turkey

- 1 lb ground turkey
- 1 15-oz can kidney or pinto beans, drained and rinsed
- 1 can low-fat, low-sodium chicken broth
- 1 14.5-oz can diced tomatoes, undrained (flavored with chilies if you can find it)
- 1 6-oz can tomato paste
- 1 Tbsp chili powder
- 1/8 tsp cinnamon
- 1/4 tsp cumin
- 1/2 tsp fresh ground black pepper

1. In a large nonstick saucepan, brown the ground turkey until it is no longer pink. Drain off any excess fat.

2. Add the remaining ingredients and bring to a boil. Lower the heat and simmer for 10 minutes.

Exchanges

2 Starch
4 Very Lean Meat

Calories 293
  Calories from Fat . . 47
Total Fat . . . . 5 g
  Saturated Fat . . . . . . 0 g
Cholesterol . . . . 63 mg
Sodium . . . . 596 mg
Carbohydrate . . . . . . 30 g
  Dietary Fiber . . . . . . 8 g
  Sugars . . . . 7 g
Protein . . . . 33 g

Southwestern Dinner Torta

Serves 4   Serving size: 1/4 torta
Preparation time: 20 minutes   Cooking time: 55 minutes

SHELF-STABLE FOODS: broth, crushed tomatoes, spices, canned beans

ALSO VISIT: meat department for turkey; salad bar for green onions; refrigerated section for tortillas, cheese

1/2	lb ground turkey or chicken
3	Tbsp low-fat, low-sodium chicken broth
1	cup diced onion
2	medium red bell peppers, cored, seeded, and thinly sliced
1	14-oz can crushed tomatoes
1	Tbsp chili powder
1	tsp cumin
1/4	tsp oregano
1/4	tsp fresh ground black pepper
	Pinch cayenne
1	15-oz can pinto or kidney beans, drained and rinsed
4	10-inch whole-wheat tortillas
1/2	cup sliced green onions
1/2	cup shredded fat-free cheddar cheese

Exchanges
4 Starch
1 Vegetable
2 Lean Meat

Calories 459
　Calories from Fat . . 60
Total Fat . . . . 7 g
　Saturated Fat . . . . . . 1 g
Cholesterol . . . . 33 mg
Sodium . . . . 975 mg
Carbohydrate . . . . . . 68 g
　Dietary Fiber . . . . . 13 g
　Sugars . . . . 13 g
Protein . . . . 32 g

1. Preheat oven to 350°F. In a large nonstick skillet over medium-high heat, sauté ground meat for 5–6 minutes. Drain fat. Add broth, onion, and peppers. Sauté 5 minutes. Add crushed tomatoes, chili powder, cumin, oregano, and pepper. Bring to a boil. Lower the heat and simmer 20 minutes.

2. Spray bottom of a springform pan with nonstick cooking spray. Layer 1 tortilla, 1/2 beans, 1 tortilla, 1/2 turkey, and repeat. Top with green onions. Bake for 20 minutes. Add cheese and bake another 5 minutes. Remove from oven. Carefully remove spring from the pan and remove ring. Cut into wedges and serve.

Crispy Rice Crust Quiche

Serves 4   Serving size: 1/4 quiche
Preparation time: 10 minutes
Cooking time: 35 minutes

SHELF-STABLE FOODS: rice, spices

ALSO VISIT: dairy case for eggs, Parmesan cheese, egg substitute, milk; salad bar for tomatoes

2 cups cooked brown rice (either instant or regular)

1 egg white or 2 Tbsp egg substitute

2 Tbsp grated Parmesan cheese

1 tsp oregano

1/4 tsp basil

1/4 tsp fresh ground black pepper

1/4 tsp salt

Egg substitute equivalent to 4 eggs

2/3 cup low-fat milk

Pinch nutmeg

1/4 cup fresh grated Parmesan cheese

1 large tomato, sliced

1. Preheat oven to 375°F. Combine the rice, egg white, Parmesan cheese, oregano, basil, pepper, and salt. Press into the bottom and up the sides of a 9-inch nonstick pie plate (or a Pyrex pie plate sprayed with nonstick spray). Bake the rice crust for 5 minutes. Remove from the oven.

2. Combine the eggs, milk, nutmeg, and Parmesan cheese. Mix well. Pour into the rice crust. Lower the oven to 350°. Bake quiche for 25 minutes.

3. Add tomatoes in a circle on top of the egg filling. Continue to bake until filling is set or a knife inserted near the center comes out clean and tomatoes are slightly browned, about 5–6 minutes.

Exchanges

2 Starch
1 Lean Meat

Calories 220
    Calories from Fat . . 44
Total Fat . . . . 5 g
    Saturated Fat . . . . . . 3 g
Cholesterol . . . . 13 mg
Sodium . . . . 490 mg
Carbohydrate . . . . . . 29 g
    Dietary Fiber . . . . . . 2 g
    Sugars . . . . 5 g
Protein . . . . 16 g

Jasmine Rice Shrimp Cakes

Serves 4   Serving size: 1 cake
Preparation time: 10 minutes
Cooking time: 10 minutes
Standing time: 15 minutes

SHELF-STABLE FOODS: jasmine rice, flour, soy sauce, breadcrumbs, spices, canned shrimp

ALSO VISIT: salad bar for green onions; dairy case for eggs; produce for garlic

2	cups cooked jasmine rice (or use regular white or brown rice)
1	egg
1 1/2	Tbsp flour
2	Tbsp finely minced green onions
1	clove garlic, finely minced
1	cup minced cooked shrimp (either canned and drained or fresh cooked, shelled and deveined)
2	tsp lite soy sauce
1	Tbsp plain breadcrumbs
1/4	tsp salt
1/4	tsp fresh ground black pepper
2	tsp canola oil

1. In a large bowl, combine all the ingredients except the oil.

2. Form the mixture into four patties. Let the patties rest for 15 minutes on a plate in the refrigerator.

3. In a large nonstick skillet over medium-high heat, heat the oil. Add the cakes and cook for about 4–5 minutes per side or until golden brown. Drain on paper toweling.

Exchanges
2 Starch
1 Very Lean Meat

Calories 195
  Calories from Fat . . 39
Total Fat . . . . 4 g
  Saturated Fat . . . . . . 1 g
Cholesterol . . . . 96 mg
Sodium . . . . 320 mg
Carbohydrate . . . . . . 27 g
  Dietary Fiber . . . . . . 1 g
  Sugars . . . . 1 g
Protein . . . . 10 g

Cinnamon Rice Pilaf

Serves 6   Serving size: 1 cup
Preparation time: 15 minutes
Cooking time: 36 minutes

SHELF-STABLE FOODS: rice, broth, raisins, cashews, spices

ALSO VISIT: salad bar for onion; produce for garlic; frozen foods for peas

- 2 tsp canola oil
- 1 large onion, diced
- 1 clove garlic, minced
- 1 cinnamon stick
- 2 whole cloves
- 1 large red bell pepper, cut into matchsticks
- 1 cup raw white rice or basmati rice
- 1 Tbsp curry powder
- 2 cups low-fat, low-sodium chicken broth
- 1 10-oz pkg frozen peas
- 1/2 cup golden raisins
- 2 Tbsp toasted cashews
- Salt and fresh ground pepper to taste

1. In a large skillet over medium-high heat, heat the oil. Add the onion, garlic, cinnamon stick, and cloves and sauté for 4 minutes, stirring occasionally.

2. Add the red bell pepper and sauté for 3 minutes. Add the rice and curry powder and sauté for 4 minutes.

3. Add the broth and bring to a boil. Lower the heat to low, cover, and simmer for 15–20 minutes. Add the peas, raisins, and cashews and simmer for 5 more minutes. Stir in salt and pepper to taste. Remove the cinnamon stick and cloves before serving.

Exchanges
2 1/2 Starch
1/2 Fruit

Calories 248
    Calories from Fat . . 31
Total Fat . . . . 3 g
    Saturated Fat . . . . . . 0 g
Cholesterol . . . . 0 mg
Sodium . . . . 283 mg
Carbohydrate . . . . . . 48 g
    Dietary Fiber . . . . . . 5 g
    Sugars . . . . 14 g
Protein . . . . 8 g

Crazy Mixed-Up Rice

Serves 6   Serving size: 1 cup
Preparation time: 15 minutes
Cooking time: 31 minutes

SHELF-STABLE FOODS: rice, spices, broth, canned beans

ALSO VISIT: salad bar for onions, red pepper; produce for garlic, cilantro; meat department for sausage

2	tsp canola oil
1/2	cup diced onion
1	clove garlic, minced
1	14-oz pkg cooked low-fat turkey sausage, sliced
1	large red bell pepper, thinly sliced
1	cup raw rice
1	Tbsp chili powder
2	cups low-fat, low-sodium chicken broth
1/2	cup frozen corn
1/2	cup canned kidney beans, rinsed and drained
1	Tbsp minced cilantro
	Salt and fresh ground black pepper to taste

1. In a skillet over medium-high heat, heat the oil. Add the onion, garlic, and turkey sausage and sauté for 5 minutes. Remove the sausage from the skillet.

2. Add the red bell pepper to the skillet and sauté for 3 minutes. Add the rice and sauté for 2 minutes. Add the chili powder and sauté for 1 minute.

3. Return the sausage to the skillet. Add the broth and bring to a boil. Lower the heat and simmer for 15 minutes. Add the corn and kidney beans and simmer for 5 more minutes until rice is tender. Add cilantro, salt, and pepper.

Exchanges
2 1/2 Starch
1 Lean Meat

Calories 269
  Calories from Fat . . 46
Total Fat . . . . 5 g
  Saturated Fat . . . . . . 1 g
Cholesterol . . . . 28 mg
Sodium . . . . 802 mg
Carbohydrate . . . . . . 41 g
  Dietary Fiber . . . . . . 2 g
  Sugars . . . . 5 g
Protein . . . . 13 g

Arroz Con Pollo Salad

Serves 4   Serving size: 3 oz chicken, 1/2 cup rice, 1/2 cup peas
Preparation time: 20 minutes
Standing time: 50 minutes

SHELF-STABLE FOODS: bottled lemon juice, saffron, spices, rice, olives, pimento

ALSO VISIT: deli for chicken; frozen foods for peas; salad bar for red onion, lettuce

1 1/2	Tbsp olive oil
2	Tbsp lemon juice
2	large pinches saffron threads
2	Tbsp warm water
1	clove garlic, minced
1/4	tsp paprika
1/4	tsp oregano
1/4	tsp crushed red pepper
1/8	tsp salt and fresh ground black pepper
12	oz cubed cooked chicken
2	cups cooked rice
2	cups frozen cooked peas
1/2	cup thinly sliced red onion
1/2	cup sliced black olives
1/4	cup chopped pimento
	Romaine lettuce leaves

Exchanges

2 1/2 Starch
3 Lean Meat
1/2 Monounsaturated Fat

Calories 408
    Calories from Fat . 122
Total Fat . . . . 14 g
    Saturated Fat . . . . . . 3 g
Cholesterol . . . . 75 mg
Sodium . . . . 998 mg
Carbohydrate . . . . . . 38 g
    Dietary Fiber . . . . . . 6 g
    Sugars . . . . 7 g
Protein . . . . 32 g

1. In a medium bowl, combine the oil and lemon juice. In a measuring cup, dissolve the saffron in the warm water. Add to the oil and lemon juice. Add the garlic, paprika, oregano, crushed red pepper flakes, salt, and pepper. Add the chicken and marinate for 20 minutes.

2. Add the remaining ingredients to the chicken except the lettuce. Chill for 30 minutes. Serve the salad on plates lined with romaine lettuce leaves.

Old-Fashioned Corn and Rice Pudding

Serves 4   Serving size: 1 cup
Preparation time: 10 minutes
Cooking time: 45 minutes

SHELF-STABLE FOODS: rice, spices

ALSO VISIT: salad bar for onion; dairy case for cheese, milk; frozen foods for corn

      2 cups cooked rice
      1 cup cooked corn (use frozen and thawed)
    1/4 cup minced onion
      1 cup grated low-fat cheddar cheese
    3/4 cup low-fat milk
    1/4 tsp chili powder
    1/4 tsp salt and fresh ground black pepper
         Paprika

1. Preheat oven to 350°F.

2. In a large bowl, combine all the ingredients except the paprika. Pour into a 1-quart nonstick casserole or a Pyrex casserole dish coated with nonstick spray. Sprinkle top of mixture with paprika.

3. Bake for 45 minutes until pudding is set.

Exchanges
2 Starch
1 Very Lean Meat

Calories 210
   Calories from Fat . . 26
Total Fat . . . . 3 g
   Saturated Fat . . . . . . 1 g
Cholesterol . . . . 8 mg
Sodium . . . . 347 mg
Carbohydrate . . . . . . 34 g
   Dietary Fiber . . . . . . 2 g
   Sugars . . . . 4 g
Protein . . . . 12 g

Hearty Vegetable Stew with Chickpeas

Serves 6   Serving size: 1 cup
Preparation time: 20 minutes
Cooking time: 25 minutes

SHELF-STABLE FOODS: canned tomatoes, broth, chickpeas, raisins, spices, flour

ALSO VISIT: salad bar for onions, red bell pepper, carrots; produce for garlic, zucchini

2	tsp canola oil
1	cup diced onion
3	cloves garlic, minced
1/2	cup minced red bell pepper
1/2	cup sliced celery
1	cup sliced carrots
1	Tbsp flour
1/2	tsp cinnamon
1/4	tsp cumin
1/4	tsp coriander
1/8	tsp ground cloves
	Pinch crushed red pepper
1	medium zucchini, sliced
1	14.5-oz can whole tomatoes, coarsely chopped, with juices
1	cup low-fat, low-sodium vegetable or chicken broth
1	16-oz can chickpeas, drained
1/2	cup dark raisins
1/4	tsp salt
1/4	tsp fresh ground black pepper

1. In a heavy kettle or Dutch oven over medium-high heat, heat the oil. Add the onion and garlic and sauté for 3 minutes. Lower the heat to medium. Add the red bell pepper, celery, and carrots and sauté for 5 minutes.

2. Sprinkle the flour over the vegetables and sauté for 30 seconds. Add the cinnamon, cumin, coriander, cloves, and crushed red pepper. Sauté for 30 seconds.

3. Add the zucchini, canned tomatoes with their liquid, and broth. Bring to a boil, lower the heat, and simmer for 10 minutes, stirring occasionally.

4. Add the chickpeas, raisins, salt, and pepper and simmer for 5 minutes more.

Exchanges
1 Starch
1/2 Fruit
2 Vegetable
1/2 Monounsaturated Fat

Calories 186
 Calories from Fat . . 29
Total Fat . . . . 3 g
 Saturated Fat . . . . . . 0 g
Cholesterol . . . . 0 mg
Sodium . . . . 397 mg
Carbohydrate . . . . . . 35 g
 Dietary Fiber . . . . . . 7 g
 Sugars . . . . 16 g
Protein . . . . 7 g

Slimming Spanish Rice with Low-Fat Turkey Sausage

Serves 4   Serving size: 3/4 cup rice, 3/4 cup vegetables, 3–4 oz sausage
Preparation time: 15 minutes
Cooking time: 31 minutes

SHELF-STABLE FOODS: rice, broth, Mexican-style canned tomatoes, spices

ALSO VISIT: salad bar for onions, red bell pepper; meat department for sausage

2	tsp olive oil
1/2	tsp cumin
	Pinch crushed red pepper
1	cup diced onions
1	cup diced red bell pepper
2	cloves garlic, minced
1	cup raw long-grain rice
1/2	tsp oregano
1	lb sliced low-fat turkey sausage
2	cups low-fat, low-sodium chicken broth
1	14.5-oz can chopped Mexican-style tomatoes with their liquid

1. In a skillet over medium-high heat, heat the oil. Add the cumin and crushed red pepper and sauté for 1 minute. Reduce heat to medium.

2. Add the onions, bell peppers, and garlic and sauté for 5 minutes. Add the rice and sauté for 2 minutes. Add the oregano and turkey sausage and sauté for 3 minutes.

3. Add the broth and tomatoes and bring to a boil. Lower the heat and simmer for 20 minutes until rice is tender.

Exchanges
3 1/2 Starch
2 Vegetable
1 Lean Meat
1/2 Fat

Calories 407
   Calories from Fat . . 73
Total Fat . . . . 8 g
   Saturated Fat . . . . . . 3 g
Cholesterol . . . . 48 mg
Sodium . . . . 1424 mg
Carbohydrate . . . . . . 61 g
   Dietary Fiber . . . . . . 3 g
   Sugars . . . . 12 g
Protein . . . . 21 g

Italian Rice Pilaf with Sautéed Chicken

Serves 4   Serving size: 3 oz chicken, 3/4 cup rice
Preparation time: 15 minutes   Cooking time: 32 minutes

SHELF-STABLE FOODS: rice, broth, spices, white wine, pine nuts, sun-dried tomatoes

ALSO VISIT: salad bar for onion; produce for garlic, parsley, basil; meat department for chicken

2 tsp olive oil	
3 cloves garlic, minced	
1/2 cup minced onion	**Exchanges**
1 cup raw long-grain rice	3 Starch
2 cups low-fat, low-sodium chicken broth	3 Very Lean Meat 1/2 Monounsaturated Fat
1/2 tsp dried oregano	
1/4 tsp salt	**Calories** 380
1 lb boneless, skinless chicken breasts, cut into 3-inch strips	Calories from Fat . . 73 **Total Fat** . . . . 8 g Saturated Fat . . . . . . 2 g
2 Tbsp dry white wine	**Cholesterol** . . . . 68 mg
2 Tbsp toasted pine nuts	**Sodium** . . . . 521 mg
1/2 cup slivered rehydrated sun-dried tomatoes	**Carbohydrate** . . . . . . 43 g Dietary Fiber . . . . . . 2 g Sugars . . . . 4 g
2 Tbsp minced Italian parsley	**Protein** . . . . 32 g
2 Tbsp minced fresh basil	
Fresh ground pepper	

1. In a skillet over medium-high heat, heat the oil. Add the garlic and onion and sauté for 2–4 minutes. Add the rice and sauté for 1 minute. Add the broth, oregano, and salt and bring to a boil. Lower the heat, cover, and simmer for 20 minutes.

2. Meanwhile, in a skillet sprayed with nonstick spray, sauté the chicken for 5–6 minutes until no longer pink. Add the wine and cook for 1–2 minutes more. Add the pine nuts, tomatoes, parsley, and basil. Add the chicken mixture to the rice and stir to mix well. Season liberally with pepper.

Southwestern Pasta and Beans

**Serves 4   Serving size: 1 cup pasta, 1/4 cup vegetables,
1/2 cup beans**

Preparation time: 15 minutes

**Cooking time: 10 minutes (add 10–12 minutes to cook pasta if not
cooked before starting recipe)**

SHELF-STABLE FOODS: spices, canned beans, broth, pasta, salsa

ALSO VISIT: salad bar for green onions; produce for garlic, cilantro

2	tsp olive oil
1/2	cup sliced green onions
2	cloves garlic, minced
1/2	tsp chili powder
1/4	tsp cumin
1/4	tsp salt
1/4	tsp fresh ground black pepper
2	cups canned black beans, rinsed and drained
1/3	cup low-fat, low-sodium chicken broth
4	cups cooked wagon-wheel pasta
1/2	cup canned salsa

Garnish: 2 Tbsp minced cilantro

1. In a skillet over medium heat, heat the oil. Add the green onions and garlic and sauté for 3 minutes. Add the chili powder, cumin, and pepper and stir to coat onions and garlic.

2. Add the beans and broth and simmer for 5 minutes.

3. Add the pasta and salsa and cook through for 1 minute. Garnish with cilantro.

Exchanges

3 1/2 Starch
1 Vegetable

Calories 301
    Calories from Fat . . 25
Total Fat . . . . 3 g
    Saturated Fat . . . . . 10 g
Cholesterol . . . . 0 mg
Sodium . . . . 565 mg
Carbohydrate . . . . . . 55 g
    Dietary Fiber . . . . . 10 g
    Sugars . . . . 7 g
Protein . . . . 13 g

Creamy Fettuccine with Artichokes and Olives

Serves 4   Serving size: 1 cup pasta, 1/2 cup artichokes
Preparation time: 10 minutes
Cooking time: 10 minutes (add 10 minutes to cook fettuccine if not cooked before starting recipe)

SHELF-STABLE FOODS: evaporated fat-free milk, artichoke hearts, capers, black olives, flour, fettuccine

ALSO VISIT: salad bar for onion, green onion; produce for garlic, parsley; dairy case for Parmesan cheese

2 tsp olive oil

1 medium onion, diced

2 cloves garlic, minced

2 green onions, sliced

2 Tbsp all-purpose flour

1 12-oz can evaporated fat-free milk

1/4 tsp salt

1/4 tsp ground black pepper

Pinch nutmeg

2 14-oz cans artichoke hearts, drained and cut in half

2 Tbsp capers

1/2 cup sliced black olives

4 cups cooked fettuccine

Exchanges
3 Starch
1 Fat Free Milk
1 Vegetable
1 1/2 Monounsaturated Fat

Calories 425
  Calories from Fat . 112
Total Fat . . . . 12 g
  Saturated Fat . . . . . . 3 g
Cholesterol . . . . 48 mg
Sodium . . . . 1184 mg
Carbohydrate . . . . . . 62 g
  Dietary Fiber . . . . . . 5 g
  Sugars . . . . 15 g
Protein . . . . 21 g

Garnish: 1/4 cup fresh grated Parmesan cheese, 1/4 cup minced parsley

1. In a skillet over medium-high heat, heat the oil. Add the onion, garlic, and green onion and sauté for 4 minutes, stirring frequently.

2. Sprinkle the flour over the onion mixture and cook 20 seconds. Add the milk, salt, pepper, and nutmeg and cook until thickened.

3. Add the artichoke hearts, capers, and olives to the sauce and cook 1 minute. Toss the sauce with the cooked fettuccine. Sprinkle each serving with cheese and parsley.

Smoky Penne Pasta

Serves 4   Serving size: 1 cup pasta, 1/2 cup sauce
Preparation time: 10 minutes
**Cooking time: 30 minutes (add 10 minutes to cook penne if not
cooked before starting recipe)**

SHELF-STABLE FOODS: canned plum tomatoes, spices, penne pasta

ALSO VISIT: deli or meat department for smoked ham or Canadian bacon; refrigerated section for Romano cheese; produce for garlic

- 2   tsp olive oil
- 2   cloves garlic, minced
- 2   Tbsp minced smoked ham or Canadian bacon
- 1   16-oz can plum tomatoes, chopped, in juices
- 1/4   tsp red pepper flakes
- 4   cups cooked penne pasta

Garnish: 1/4 cup grated Romano cheese

1. In a skillet over medium heat, heat the oil. Add the garlic and ham and sauté for 5 minutes, stirring frequently.

2. Add the tomatoes and red pepper flakes and cook over medium-high heat for 5 minutes. Lower the heat and let the sauce simmer for 20 minutes or until thickened.

3. Toss the sauce with the cooked penne and top each serving with cheese.

Exchanges
2 1/2 Starch
1 Vegetable
1 Fat

Calories 278
    Calories from Fat . . 51
Total Fat . . . . 6 g
    Saturated Fat . . . . . . 2 g
Cholesterol . . . . 10 mg
Sodium . . . . 322 mg
Carbohydrate . . . . . . 46 g
    Dietary Fiber . . . . . . 3 g
    Sugars . . . . 5 g
Protein . . . . 11 g

No-Cook Peanut Pasta

Serves 4   Serving size: 1 cup pasta, 2 Tbsp sauce
Preparation time: 10 minutes
Cooking time: 0 (add 10 minutes if linguine is not cooked before starting recipe)

SHELF-STABLE FOODS: peanut butter, soy sauce, rice vinegar, sugar, hoisin sauce, linguine

ALSO VISIT: salad bar for green onions; produce for garlic

Sauce:
1/3 cup hot water

1/3 cup reduced-fat creamy peanut butter

1 Tbsp lite soy sauce

1 Tbsp rice vinegar

1 tsp sugar

2 tsp minced green onions

2 cloves garlic, finely minced

1 tsp hoisin sauce

4 cups hot cooked linguine

Combine all ingredients for the sauce and toss with hot cooked linguine.

Exchanges
3 1/2 Starch
1 Fat

Calories 329
   Calories from Fat . . 75
Total Fat . . . . 8 g
   Saturated Fat . . . . . . 1 g
Cholesterol . . . . 0 mg
Sodium . . . . 279 mg
Carbohydrate . . . . . . 56 g
   Dietary Fiber . . . . . . 4 g
   Sugars . . . . 7 g
Protein . . . . 12 g

Caesar Pasta with Pan-Seared Salmon

Serves 4   Serving size: 1/2 cup pasta, 1 cup vegetables, 3 oz salmon
Preparation time: 15 minutes
Cooking time: 20 minutes

SHELF-STABLE FOODS: rotini pasta, salad dressing, pesto

ALSO VISIT: salad bar for onion; produce for garlic; frozen foods for green bean and carrot blend; refrigerated section for Parmesan cheese; seafood department for salmon

1 tsp olive oil	
2 cloves garlic, minced	
1 small onion, minced	
1 lb fresh salmon, cut into 2-inch cubes	
8 oz uncooked rotini pasta	
4 cups frozen green bean and carrot blend	
1/2 cup fat-free or reduced-fat Caesar salad dressing	
1 Tbsp prepared pesto	
1/4 tsp fresh ground black pepper	

Garnish: 1/4 cup fresh grated Parmesan cheese

Exchanges

3 Starch
3 Vegetable
3 Lean Meat
1 Fat

Calories 540
   Calories from Fat . 136
Total Fat . . . . 15 g
   Saturated Fat . . . . . . 5 g
Cholesterol . . . . 86 mg
Sodium . . . . 590 mg
Carbohydrate . . . . . . 62 g
   Dietary Fiber . . . . . . 6 g
   Sugars . . . . 11 g
Protein . . . . 37 g

1. In a nonstick skillet over medium heat, heat the oil. Add the garlic and onions and cook for 4 minutes. Add the salmon and cook over medium-high heat until salmon is seared on all sides, about 5–6 minutes. Set aside.

2. Meanwhile, bring a pot of water to a boil. Add the pasta and cook for 5–6 minutes. Add the frozen vegetables, return to a boil, and cook for 3 more minutes until vegetables are done and pasta is cooked al dente. Drain.

3. In a large bowl, toss the pasta mixture with the salmon. Add the Caesar dressing, pesto, and pepper and mix well. Serve at room temperature or allow mixture to chill for 30 minutes in the refrigerator.

4. Top each serving with fresh grated cheese.

The Fastest Stir-Fry Pasta

Serves 4   Serving size: 1 cup pasta, 1 cup vegetables, 3 oz chicken
Preparation time: 10 minutes
Cooking time: 15 minutes

SHELF-STABLE FOODS: lo mein noodles or fettuccine, soy sauce, hoisin sauce, broth, ground ginger

ALSO VISIT: meat department for chicken; frozen foods for stir-fry vegetables

1	lb boneless, skinless chicken tenders or cubed chicken breasts
1/4	cup lite soy sauce
2	tsp sesame oil
2	Tbsp hoisin sauce
1/2	cup low-fat, low-sodium chicken broth
1/4	tsp ground ginger
4	cups frozen stir-fry vegetables
	Pinch crushed red pepper
4	cups cooked lo mein noodles or fettuccine

1. In a large nonstick skillet or a wok sprayed with cooking spray, stir-fry the chicken over medium-high heat for about 5–6 minutes.

2. Combine the soy sauce, sesame oil, hoisin sauce, broth, ginger, and crushed red pepper in a measuring cup. Add to the chicken. Add the frozen vegetables and cover and steam until vegetables are crisp, yet tender, about 5–9 minutes.

3. Serve the mixture over the cooked noodles.

Exchanges

3 Starch
2 Vegetable
3 Very Lean Meat

Calories	393
Calories from Fat	46
Total Fat	5 g
Saturated Fat	1 g
Cholesterol	68 mg
Sodium	913 mg
Carbohydrate	51 g
Dietary Fiber	4 g
Sugars	8 g
Protein	32 g

Spiced Pork and Broccoli with Lo Mein Noodles

Serves 4   Serving size: 1 cup pasta, 1 cup vegetables, 3 oz pork
Preparation time: 15 minutes
Cooking time: 15 minutes (add 6–8 minutes for lo mein noodles if not cooked before starting recipe)

SHELF-STABLE FOODS: spices, broth, soy sauce, sherry or rice vinegar, lo mein noodles, sesame oil

ALSO VISIT: meat department for pork; salad bar for mushrooms, broccoli, bean sprouts

1	lb boneless pork loin, cut into 2-inch strips
1	tsp cinnamon
2	tsp garlic powder
1	tsp onion powder
1/2	tsp ginger
1/4	tsp chili powder
1/8	tsp salt
1/4	tsp fresh ground black pepper
1	tsp sesame oil
2	cups sliced mushrooms
1/4	cup low-fat, low-sodium chicken broth
2	Tbsp lite soy sauce
1	Tbsp dry sherry or rice vinegar
2	cups broccoli florets
4	cups cooked lo mein noodles or spaghetti
1	cup fresh bean sprouts (optional)

1. In a zippered plastic bag, combine the pork strips with the cinnamon, garlic powder, onion powder, ground ginger, chili powder, salt, and pepper. Shake until pork is coated. Set aside for 5 minutes.

2. In a large wok over medium-high heat, heat the oil. Add the mushrooms and stir-fry for 3 minutes. Add the pork strips and stir-fry for 7–8 minutes until the pork is cooked through.

3. Combine the broth, soy sauce, and sherry. Add to the wok. Add the broccoli. Cover and steam for 3–4 minutes on low heat.

4. Serve the pork and broccoli over the cooked lo mein noodles and top with bean sprouts if desired.

Exchanges

3 Starch
1 Vegetable
3 Very Lean Meat

Calories 372
  Calories from Fat . . 59
Total Fat . . . . 7 g
  Saturated Fat . . . . . . 2 g
Cholesterol . . . . 64 mg
Sodium . . . . 470 mg
Carbohydrate . . . . . . 49 g
  Dietary Fiber . . . . . . 4 g
  Sugars . . . . 4 g
Protein . . . . 32 g

Cheesy Bow Ties with Asparagus and Carrots

Serves 4   Serving size: 1 cup pasta, 1 cup vegetables, 1/2 cup cheese sauce

Preparation time: 15 minutes

Cooking time: 17 minutes (includes cooking the pasta if not already prepared)

SHELF-STABLE FOODS: pasta, broth, spices

ALSO VISIT: produce or salad bar for asparagus, carrots, onion; dairy case for margarine, ricotta cheese, cottage cheese, feta cheese, Parmesan cheese

- 2 Tbsp reduced-fat margarine
- 2 cups sliced asparagus (1 1/2-inch slices)
- 2 cups thinly sliced carrots
- 2 cloves garlic, minced
- 1/4 cup minced onion
- 1 cup fat-free ricotta cheese
- 1 cup low-fat cottage cheese
- 1/3 cup fresh grated Parmesan cheese
- 1 Tbsp crumbled feta cheese
- 2 Tbsp low-fat, low-sodium chicken broth
- 1 tsp dried oregano
- 1/8 tsp salt
- 1/4 tsp fresh ground black pepper
- 4 cups cooked bow tie pasta

Exchanges

2 1/2 Starch
2 Vegetable
2 Lean Meat

Calories	370
Calories from Fat	68
Total Fat	8 g
Saturated Fat	2 g
Cholesterol	31 mg
Sodium	510 mg
Carbohydrate	51 g
Dietary Fiber	5 g
Sugars	13 g
Protein	27 g

1. In a large skillet over medium-high heat, heat the margarine. Add the asparagus, carrots, onion, and garlic and sauté for 5–7 minutes.

2. Reduce the heat to medium. Add the ricotta cheese, cottage cheese, Parmesan cheese, feta cheese, and broth. Stir well to combine. Add the oregano, salt, and pepper.

3. Toss the mixture with hot cooked bow tie pasta.

All White Bean Salad

Serves 4 Serving size: 1/2 cup
Preparation time: 15 minutes
Standing time: several hours

SHELF-STABLE FOODS: canned beans, vinegar

ALSO VISIT: salad bar for green onions, celery; produce for parsley

- 1 cup cannelini beans, rinsed and drained
- 1 cup navy beans, rinsed and drained
- 1/2 cup minced green onions
- 1/2 cup minced Italian parsley
- 1/4 cup minced celery
- 2 Tbsp balsamic vinegar
- 1 Tbsp olive oil
- Fresh ground pepper

Combine all ingredients in a salad bowl and refrigerate for several hours.

Exchanges
2 Starch
1/2 Monounsaturated Fat

Calories 172
   Calories from Fat . . 36
Total Fat . . . . 4 g
   Saturated Fat . . . . . . 1 g
Cholesterol . . . . 0 mg
Sodium . . . . 209 mg
Carbohydrate . . . . . . 27 g
   Dietary Fiber . . . . . . 7 g
   Sugars . . . . 4 g
Protein . . . . 8 g

Pasta, Kale, and White Bean Ragout

Serves 4   Serving size: 1 cup pasta, 1 cup vegetables and beans
Preparation time: 10 minutes
Cooking time: 15 minutes

SHELF-STABLE FOODS: pasta, Italian salad dressing, beans, olives

ALSO VISIT: frozen foods for kale; salad bar for onion, tomatoes; dairy case for Parmesan cheese; produce for basil

2 tsp olive oil

1 small onion, diced

2 cloves garlic, minced

1 10-oz pkg frozen chopped kale, thawed

1 15-oz can white beans, drained

1 cup diced tomatoes

1/4 cup sliced green olives

2 Tbsp chopped basil

2/3 cup fat-free Italian salad dressing

2 Tbsp grated Parmesan cheese

4 cups cooked ziti pasta

1. In a skillet over medium heat, heat the oil. Add the onion and garlic and sauté for 3–5 minutes. Add the kale and sauté for 2–3 minutes. Add the beans, tomatoes, olives, and basil and sauté for 2 minutes.

2. Add the salad dressing, Parmesan cheese, and ziti. Cook for 1–2 minutes more.

Exchanges
4 Starch
1 Vegetable
1/2 Monounsaturated Fat

Calories 380
  Calories from Fat . . 57
Total Fat . . . . 6 g
  Saturated Fat . . . . . . 1 g
Cholesterol . . . . 4 mg
Sodium . . . . 846 mg
Carbohydrate . . . . . . 65 g
  Dietary Fiber . . . . . . 9 g
  Sugars . . . . 11 g
Protein . . . . 16 g

Vegetable Chili

Serves 5   Serving size: 1 cup
Preparation time: 20 minutes
Cooking time: 1 hour

SHELF-STABLE FOODS: tomatoes, broth, tomato sauce, black beans, spices

ALSO VISIT: salad bar (or produce) for onion, cabbage

1	Tbsp olive oil
1	cup diced onion
3	cloves garlic, minced
2	cups chopped green cabbage
1	28-oz can tomatoes, coarsely chopped, drained and 1 cup liquid reserved
1	cup low-fat, low-sodium chicken broth
1	8-oz can tomato sauce
1	15-oz can black beans, drained and rinsed
2	Tbsp chili powder
1	bay leaf
1	tsp cumin
1/4	tsp cayenne pepper
	Fresh ground pepper and salt to taste

1. In a large stockpot over medium heat, heat the oil. Add the onion and garlic and sauté for 5 minutes.

2. Add remaining ingredients. Bring to a boil. Lower the heat and simmer for 1 hour until thick. Add reserved tomato liquid as necessary. Remove bay leaf before serving.

Exchanges
1 Starch
3 Vegetable
1/2 Monounsaturated Fat

Calories 165
    Calories from Fat . . 35
Total Fat . . . . 4 g
    Saturated Fat . . . . . . 1 g
Cholesterol . . . . 0 mg
Sodium . . . . 725 mg
Carbohydrate . . . . . . 28 g
    Dietary Fiber . . . . . . 9 g
    Sugars . . . . 11 g
Protein . . . . 8 g

Pasta and White Bean Casserole

Serves 6   Serving size: 3–4 oz turkey, 1 cup pasta,
1 cup vegetables and beans
Preparation time: 25 minutes

SHELF-STABLE FOODS: tomatoes, broth, beans, pasta, breadcrumbs

ALSO VISIT: meat department for turkey; salad bar for broccoli, onion; dairy case for Parmesan cheese

1 1/2 lb ground turkey

1 small onion, diced

2 cups chopped broccoli

1 tsp dry sage

1 tsp dry tarragon

1 16-oz can tomatoes, liquid reserved, finely chopped

1 1/2 cups low-fat, low-sodium chicken broth

1 15-oz can white beans, drained

6 cups cooked Rotini pasta

2 Tbsp plain breadcrumbs

2 Tbsp Parmesan cheese

Exchanges

4 Starch
1 Vegetable
4 Very Lean Meat

Calories 492
   Calories from Fat . . 59
Total Fat . . . . 7 g
   Saturated Fat . . . . . . 1 g
Cholesterol . . . . 65 mg
Sodium . . . . 431 mg
Carbohydrate . . . . . . 67 g
   Dietary Fiber . . . . . . 7 g
   Sugars . . . . 6 g
Protein . . . . 39 g

1. Preheat oven to 350°F. Crumble turkey into a large skillet and place over medium heat. Cook, stirring occasionally, until turkey is cooked through, about 4–5 minutes. Pour off all but 1 Tbsp of the drippings from the skillet.

2. Add onion, broccoli, sage, and tarragon to skillet. Cook until vegetables are soft, about 4 minutes. (Note: The broccoli may not be soft yet, but it will be after baking.)

3. Add tomatoes and heat to boiling, stirring occasionally. Boil 3 minutes. Remove skillet from heat and add chicken broth, reserved tomato liquid, and beans. Stir well.

4. In a large bowl, combine broccoli mixture and turkey with cooked pasta. Toss well. Transfer mixture to a baking dish coated with nonstick spray. Combine crumbs with cheese. Sprinkle over casserole. Bake until heated through, about 20 minutes.

Baked Rotini with Chickpea-Tomato Sauce

Serves 8   Serving size: 1/8 recipe
Preparation time: 20 minutes   Cooking time: 30 minutes

SHELF-STABLE FOODS: chickpeas, tomatoes, tomato juice, noodles, breadcrumbs, sesame seeds

ALSO VISIT: salad bar for green onions; produce for garlic; dairy case for yogurt

2   15-oz cans chickpeas, drained and rinsed

1   18-oz can crushed tomatoes

1 1/4   cups spicy tomato juice

2   cloves garlic, minced

6   green onions, thinly sliced, green and white parts separated

1   tsp cumin

Fresh ground pepper and salt to taste

1/3   cup plain fat-free yogurt

6   cups cooked rotini noodles, undercooked by 3 minutes

1/2   cup plain dry breadcrumbs

1   Tbsp sesame seeds

1   Tbsp olive oil

Exchanges
4 Starch
2 Vegetable
1/2 Fat

Calories 396
  Calories from Fat . . 60
Total Fat . . . . 7 g
  Saturated Fat . . . . . . 1 g
Cholesterol . . . . 0 mg
Sodium . . . . 481 mg
Carbohydrate . . . . . . 69 g
  Dietary Fiber . . . . . . 9 g
  Sugars . . . . 11 g
Protein . . . . 15 g

1. Preheat oven to 375°F. Combine chickpeas, tomatoes, juice, garlic, white parts of green onions, cumin, pepper, and salt in a medium saucepan. Heat to boiling. Reduce heat, cover, and simmer for 10 minutes.

2. In a small bowl, slowly whisk about 1/4 cup of the tomato liquid into the yogurt. Stir the yogurt mixture into the chickpeas. Stir in the cooked pasta and toss to coat. Transfer to a baking dish.

3. Mix remaining ingredients in a small bowl until blended. Sprinkle the mixture evenly over the top of the pasta. Bake until edges are bubbly and the top is golden brown, about 15 minutes.

Fruited Couscous

Serves 6   Serving size: 1/2 cup couscous, 1/4 cup dried fruit
Preparation time: 15 minutes

SHELF-STABLE FOODS: couscous, raisins, apricots, spices, apple juice

        1 1/2 cups water

        1 1/2 cups unsweetened apple juice

        1 1/2 cups couscous

          3/4 cup golden raisins

          3/4 cup diced dried apricots

            2 tsp cinnamon

          1/2 tsp nutmeg

          1/4 tsp allspice

            2 tsp honey

1. In a medium saucepot, bring the water and apple juice to a boil. Add the couscous, raisins, and apricots. Remove from the stove and let the couscous rehydrate, uncovered, for about 5–6 minutes. Drain off any excess liquid. Couscous should be soft.

2. Add the spices and honey and serve.

Exchanges
2 Starch
2 1/2 Fruit

Calories 293
  Calories from Fat . . . 4
Total Fat . . . . 0 g
  Saturated Fat . . . . . . 0 g
Cholesterol . . . . 0 mg
Sodium . . . . 11 mg
Carbohydrate . . . . . . 67 g
  Dietary Fiber . . . . . . 4 g
  Sugars . . . . 28 g
Protein . . . . 7 g

Basil Rice Salad

Serves 6 **Serving size: 1 cup (1/2 cup rice, 1/2 cup vegetables and beans)**

Preparation time: 20 minutes

Standing time: 1–2 hours

SHELF-STABLE FOODS: rice, kidney beans, vinegar

ALSO VISIT: salad bar for carrots, tomatoes, green onions; produce for basil, parsley

3	cups cooked rice
1/2	cup diced carrots
2	medium tomatoes, diced
1	cup canned kidney beans, drained
2	green onions, minced

Dressing:

2	Tbsp lemon juice
2	Tbsp red wine vinegar
1/4	cup olive oil
1/4	cup minced basil
2	Tbsp minced Italian parsley
2	tsp sugar
	Fresh ground pepper and salt to taste

1. Combine the salad ingredients in a large bowl.

2. In a separate bowl, whisk together the dressing ingredients.

3. Add dressing to salad and toss well. Chill for 1–2 hours. Serve cold.

Exchanges

2 Starch
1 Vegetable
1 1/2 Monounsaturated Fat

Calories 246
   Calories from Fat . . 85
Total Fat . . . . 9 g
   Saturated Fat . . . . . . 2 g
Cholesterol . . . . 0 mg
Sodium . . . . 60 mg
Carbohydrate . . . . . . 35 g
   Dietary Fiber . . . . . . 3 g
   Sugars . . . . 4 g
Protein . . . . 5 g

Artichoke Tomato Lasagna

Serves 4   Serving size: 1/4 recipe
Preparation time: 35 minutes
Cooking time: 30 minutes
Standing time: 15–20 minutes

SHELF-STABLE FOODS: lasagna noodles, spices, Worcestershire sauce, crushed tomatoes, tomato paste, artichoke hearts

ALSO VISIT: salad bar for onions; dairy case for cottage cheese, ricotta, mozzarella, Parmesan

2	tsp olive oil
1	cup chopped onion
2	cloves garlic, minced
1	28-oz can crushed tomatoes
1	6-oz can tomato paste
2	tsp dried oregano leaves
1	tsp ground cumin
1	tsp dried basil leaves
2	tsp Worcestershire sauce
3/4	cup cottage cheese
3/4	cup low-fat ricotta cheese
1	cup part-skim mozzarella cheese
1/2	cup Parmesan cheese, divided
1	14-oz can artichoke hearts, packed in water, diced
9	cooked lasagna noodles

1. Preheat oven to 375°F. In a large skillet over medium heat, heat the oil. Add the onion and garlic and sauté for about 5 minutes.

2. Add the crushed tomatoes, tomato paste, oregano, cumin, basil, and Worcestershire sauce and cook over low heat for 15 minutes.

3. Meanwhile, in a large bowl, combine the cottage, ricotta, and mozzarella cheeses and half of the Parmesan cheese. Add the artichokes.

4. Dab some of the sauce over the bottom of a Pyrex baking dish. Place some of the cooked lasagna noodles over the sauce. Layer the cheese mixture on top of the noodles and layer more sauce. Continue to layer

until you have three layers, ending with sauce. Sprinkle with remaining Parmesan.

5. Cover with foil and bake for about 30 minutes. Remove cover and bake 5 minutes more. Let stand for 15–20 minutes before slicing.

Exchanges
4 Starch
6 Vegetable
2 Lean Meat
1 Saturated Fat

Calories 632
   Calories from Fat . 150
Total Fat . . . . 17 g
   Saturated Fat . . . . . . 9 g
Cholesterol . . . . 56 mg
Sodium . . . . 1404 mg
Carbohydrate . . . . . . 85 g
   Dietary Fiber . . . . . 10 g
   Sugars . . . . 20 g
Protein . . . . 40 g

Chickpea Rice Salad

Serves 6 Serving size: 1 cup rice, 1/2 cup vegetables and beans
Preparation time: 15 minutes
Cooking time: 20 minutes (to cook the rice)

SHELF-STABLE FOODS: rice, chickpeas, vinegar, oil

ALSO VISIT: salad bar for tomatoes, green onions; frozen foods for green beans

> 4 cups water
> 2 cups raw rice
> 1/2 cup frozen green beans, thawed
> 2 small ripe tomatoes, diced
> 1/2 cup minced green onions
> 3 Tbsp red wine vinegar
> 3 Tbsp olive oil
> 1 cup canned chickpeas, rinsed and drained

1. In a saucepan over high heat, bring the water to a boil. Slowly add the rice. Cover and lower the heat to simmer. Cook for 20 minutes.

2. In a large salad bowl, combine remaining ingredients. Add the cooked rice and refrigerate for several hours or serve at room temperature.

Exchanges
4 Starch
1/2 Monounsaturated Fat

Calories 344
 Calories from Fat . . 72
Total Fat . . . . 8 g
 Saturated Fat . . . . . . 2 g
Cholesterol . . . . 0 mg
Sodium . . . . 48 mg
Carbohydrate . . . . . . 60 g
 Dietary Fiber . . . . . . 4 g
 Sugars . . . . 3 g
Protein . . . . 7 g

Index

Alphabetical List of Recipes

Subject Index

Books from the American Diabetes Association

Cooking and Nutrition

NEW!

Cooking with the Diabetic Chef
Chris Smith

Introducing the first cookbook ever written for people with diabetes by a chef with diabetes! Chris Smith is living proof you can eat the foods you love and live healthy with diabetes. Pizza, chocolate, butter, burritos, sausage, veal roast, stir fry—there's virtually nothing you can't have and it all tastes great! Imagine sinking your teeth into Chocolate Chip Pancakes, Succulent Steak Teriyaki, Tender melt-in-your-mouth ribs, Dreamy chocolate cake and many more!
One Low Price: $19.95
Order #4630-01

NEW!

More Diabetic Meals in 30 Minutes—or Less!
Robyn Webb

Robyn Webb is back weaving her magic in your kitchen! She's whipped up hundreds more simply sensational recipes from mouth watering appetizers and succulent seafood dishes to tantalizing desserts. Choose from any of 225 fabulous recipes that not only satisfy your appetite and your carvings and taste savory and delicious but also meet ADA nutritional guidelines.
Each recipe gives you nutritional content and exchanges as well as fat and calorie counts.
One Low Price: $16.95
Order #4629-01

The Great Chicken Cookbook for People with Diabetes
Beryl M. Marton

Now you can have chicken any way you want it—and healthy too! More than 150 great-tasting, low-fat chicken recipes in all, including baked chicken, braised chicken, chicken casseroles, grilled chicken, rolled and stuffed chicken, chicken soups, chicken stir-fry, chicken with pasta, and many more.
One Low Price: $16.95
Order #4627-01

The New Soul Food Cookbook for People with Diabetes
Fabiola Demps Gaines, RD, LD
Roniece Weaver, RD, LD

Dig into sensational low-fat recipes from the first African American cookbook for people with diabetes. More than 150 recipes in all, including Shrimp Jambalaya, Fried Okra, Orange Sweet Potatoes, Corn Muffins, Apple Crisp, and many more.
One Low Price: $14.95
Order #4623-01

The Diabetes Snack Munch Nibble Nosh Book
Ruth Glick

Choose from 150 low-sodium, low-fat snacks and mini-meals such as Pizza Puffs, Mustard Pretzels, Apple-Cranberry Turnovers, Bread Puzzle, Cinnamon Biscuits, Pecan Buns, Alphabet Letters, Banana Pops, and many others. Special features include recipes for one or two and snack ideas for hard-to-please kids. Nutrient analyses, preparation times, and exchanges are included with every recipe.
One Low Price: $14.95
Order #4622-01

The ADA Guide to Healthy Restaurant Eating
Hope S. Warshaw, MMSc, RD, CDE

Finally! One book with all the facts you need to eat out intelligently—whether you're enjoying burgers, pizza, bagels, pasta, or burritos at your favorite restaurant. Special features include more than 2,500 menu items from more than 50 major restaurant chains, complete nutrition information for every menu item, restaurant pitfalls and strategies for defensive restaurant dining and much more.
One Low Price: $13.95
Order #4819-01

Quick & Easy Diabetic Recipes for One
Kathleen Stanley, CDE, RD, MSED
Connie C. Crawley, MS, RD, LD

More than 100 breakfast, lunch, dinner, and snack recipes cut down to single-serving size.
One Low Price: $12.95
Order #4621-01

Month of Meals: Classic Cooking

Choose from the classic tastes of Chicken Cacciatore, Oven Fried Fish, Sloppy Joes, Shish Kabobs, Roast Leg of Lamb, Lasagna, Minestrone Soup, Grilled Cheese Sandwiches, and many others. And just because it's Christmas doesn't mean you have to abandon your healthy meal plan. A Special Occasion section offers tips for brunches, holidays, parties, and

restaurants to give you delicious dining options in any setting. 58 pages.
Spiral-bound.
One Low Price: $14.95
Order #4701-01

Month of Meals: Ethnic Delights

A healthy diet doesn't have to keep you from enjoying your favorite restaurants: tips for Mexican, Italian, and Chinese restaurants are featured. Quick-to-fix and ethnic recipes are also included. Choose from Beef Burritos, Chop Suey, Veal Piccata, Stuffed Peppers, and many others. 63 pages. Spiral-bound.
One Low Price: $14.95
Order #4702-01

Month of Meals: Meals in Minutes

Eat at McDonald's, Wendy's, Taco Bell, and other fast food restaurants and still maintain a healthy diet. Special sections offer tips on planning meals when you're ill, reading ingredient labels, preparing for picnics and barbecues, more. Quick-to-fix menu choices include Seafood Stir Fry, Fajita in a Pita, Hurry-Up Beef Stew, Quick Homemade Raisin Bread, Macaroni and Cheese, many others. 80 pages. Spiral-bound.
One Low Price: $14.95
Order #4703-01

Month of Meals: Old-Time Favorites

Old-time family favorites like Meatloaf and Pot Roast will remind you of the irresistible meals grandma used to make. Hints for turning family-size meals into delicious "planned-overs" will keep leftovers from going to waste. Meal plans for one or two people are also featured. Choose from Oven Crispy Chicken, Beef Stroganoff, Kielbasa and Sauerkraut, Sausage and Cornbread Pie, and many others. 74 pages. Spiral-bound.
One Low Price: $14.95
Order #4704-01

Month of Meals: Vegetarian Pleasures

Choose from a garden of fresh selections like Eggplant Italian, Stuffed Zucchini, Cucumbers with Dill Dressing, Vegetable Lasagna, and many others. Craving a snack? Try Red Pepper Dip, Eggplant Caviar, or Beanito Spread. A special section shows you the most nutritious ways to cook with whole grains, and how to add flavor to your meals with peanuts, walnuts, pecans, pumpkin seeds, and more. 58 pages. Spiral-bound.
One Low Price: $14.95
Order #4705-01

Official Pocket Guide to Diabetic Exchanges

Finally! A pocket-sized version of ADA's most popular aid to balanced nutrition.
Nonmember: $5.95
Member: $4.95
Order #4709-01

The Diabetes Carbohydrate & Fat Gram Guide, 2nd Edition
Lea Ann Holzmeister, RD, CDE

Hundreds of charts list foods, serving sizes, and nutrient data for generic and packaged products. Now includes cholesterol, fiber, and protein.
One Low Price: $14.95
Order #4708-02

Brand-Name Diabetic Meals in Minutes

More than 200 kitchen-tested recipes from Swanson, Campbell Soup, Kraft Foods, and more.
Nonmember: $12.50
Member: $9.95
Order #4620-01

Complete Quick & Hearty Cookbook

Features dozens of simple yet delicious recipes from the best of the popular *Healthy Selects* cookbook series.
One Low Price: $12.95
Order #4624-01

BESTSELLER!

Diabetic Meals in 30 Minutes—or Less!
Robyn Webb

Choose from more than 140 delicious, quick-to-fix meals from best-selling author Robyn Webb.
Nonmember: $11.95
Member: $9.95
Order #4614-01

NEWLY REVISED BESTSELLER!

Diabetes Meal Planning Made Easy, 2nd Edition
Hope S. Warshaw, MMSc, RD, CDE

Discover how to master the food pyramid, understand Nutrition Facts and food labels, more.
One Low Price: $14.95
Order #4706-02

Magic Menus
Spanish Omelets, Blueberry Muffins, Oven-Fried Chicken, Caesar Salad, more.
Nonmember: $14.95
Member: $12.95
Order #4707-01

Memorable Menus
Robyn Webb
Roast Turkey Tenderloins, Honey-Mustard Chicken, Southern Shrimp Gumbo, more.
Nonmember: $19.95
Member: $17.95
Order #4619-01

Sweet Kids
Betty Page Brackenridge, MS, RD, CDE
Richard R. Rubin, PhD, CDE
Practical meal planning and nutrition advice for parents of diabetic children.
Nonmember: $11.95
Member: $9.95
Order #4905-01

Self-Care

NEW!

The American Diabetes Association Complete Guide to Diabetes, 2nd Edition
American Diabetes Association
Everything you ever needed to know about diabetes contained inside one practical book—now updated! One of the most complete and authoritative resources you can find on diabetes, it covers everything from how to manage types 1 and 2 and gestational diabetes to traveling with insulin, sick day action plans, and recognizing hypoglycemia. You get in-depth coverage on preventing and treating complications, recognizing symptoms, exercising, nutrition, glucose control, sexual issues, pregnancy, and more.
One Low Price: $23.95
Order #4809-02

NEW!

The Diabetes Problem Solver
Nancy Touchette, PhD
Quick: You think you may have diabetic ketoacidosis, a life-threatening condition. What are the symptoms? What should you do first? What are the

treatments? How could it have been prevented? The Diabetes Problem Solver is the first reference guide that helps you identify and prevent the most common diabetes-related problems you encounter from day to day. From hypoglycemia, nerve pain, and foot ulcers to eye disease, depression, and eating disorders, virtually every possible problem is covered. And the solutions are at your fingertips. *The Diabetes Problem Solver* addresses each problem by answering five crucial questions:

1. What are the symptoms?
2. What are the risks?
3. What do I do now?
4. What's the best treatment?
5. How can I prevent this problem?

You'll find extensive, easy-to-read coverage of just about every diabetes problem you can imagine, and comprehensive flowcharts at the front of the book lead you from symptoms to possible solutions quickly.
One Low Price: $19.95
Order #4825-01

NEW!

Diabetes Burnout: What to Do When You Can't Take It Anymore
William H. Polonsky, PhD, CDE

Living with diabetes is hard work. It's easy to get discouraged, frustrated and depressed—just plain old burned out. Finally there's a book that understands the roller-coaster of emotions you go through and gives you the tools you need to keep the "downers" from overwhelming you—all in a compassionate and even humorous way. It can help you pinpoint whether you've hit diabetes burnout (if so, you're not alone!).
One Low Price: $18.95
Order #4822-01

NEW!

16 Myths of a Diabetic Diet
Karen Hanson Chalmers, MS, RD, CDE
Amy E. Peterson, MS, RD, CDE

Now there's an easier way to debunk the myths you often hear such as "you need to eat foods sweetened with sugar substitutes instead of sugar," "don't eat too many starchy foods," and "no snacking or giving in to food cravings," even that you have to eat different food from everyone else. This exciting book sets the record straight on the 16 most common myths about food and diet.
One Low Price: $14.95
Order #4829-01

NEW!

101 Foot Care Tips for People with Diabetes
Jessie H. Ahroni, PhD, ARNP, CDE

"Diabetic foot problems cause more hospital stays than any other complication of diabetes. This book tells you what to do for good foot care. It can help you stand on your own two feet for a lifetime!"
—Neil M. Schaffler, DPM, FACFAS
President, Baltimore Podiatry Group

- What should I do if I nick myself while trimming my toenails?
- How can I tell whether my shoes fit?
- What should I do if I have bunions?

These are just a few of the 101 questions answered in this indispensable new book for people with diabetes.
One Low Price: $14.95
Order #4834-01

101 Medication Tips for People with Diabetes
Betsy A. Carlisle, PharmD
Mary Anne Koda-Kimble, PharmD, CDE
Lisa Kroon, PharmD

1. What is the difference between regular and lispro insulin?
2. What are the main side effects of the drugs used to treat type 2 diabetes?
3. Will my diabetes medications interact with other drugs I'm taking?
4. My doctor prescribed an "ACE inhibitor." What is this drug? What will it do?

Treating diabetes can get complicated, especially when you consider the bewildering number of medications that must be carefully integrated with diet and exercise. Here you'll find answers to 101 of the most commonly asked questions about diabetes and medication. An indispensable reference for anyone with type 1, type 2, or gestational diabetes.
One Low Price: $14.95
Order #4833-01

101 Nutrition Tips for People with Diabetes
Patti B. Geil, MS, RD, FADA, CDE
Lea Ann Holzmeister, RD, CDE

1. Which type of fiber helps my blood sugar?
2. What do I do if my toddler refuses to eat her meal?
3. If a food is sugar-free, can I eat all I want?

In this latest addition to the best-selling 101 Tips series, co-authors Patti Geil and Lea Ann Holzmeister—experts on nutrition and diabetes—use

their professional experience with hundreds of patients over the years to answer the most commonly asked questions about diabetes and nutrition. You'll discover handy tips on meal planning, general nutrition, managing medication and meals, shopping and cooking, weight loss, and more.
One Low Price: $14.95
Order #4828-01

NEWLY REVISED!

101 Tips for Improving Your Blood Sugar, 2nd Edition
David S. Schade, MD, and The University of New Mexico Diabetes Care Team

Last night you ate a normal meal and took your usual insulin dose. When you woke up this morning you had low blood sugar. Why?
You work hard all week and you like to reward yourself by sleeping in on weekends. How can you avoid waking up with high blood sugar?
These are just a couple of the more than 100 tips you'll discover in this newly revised second edition of an ADA bestseller. Dozens of other tips—many of them just added—will help you reduce the risk of complications from extremes in blood sugar levels.
One Low Price: $14.95
Order #4805-01

NEWLY REVISED!

101 Tips for Staying Healthy with Diabetes (& Avoiding Complications), 2nd Edition
David S. Schade, MD, and The University of New Mexico Diabetes Care Team

1. Is testing your urine for glucose and ketones an accurate way to measure blood sugar?
2. What's the best way to reduce the pain of frequent finger sticks?
3. Will an insulin pump help you prevent complications?

These are just a few of the more than 110 tips you'll discover in this newly revised second edition of an ADA bestseller. Dozens of other tips—many of them just added—will help you reduce the risk of complications and help you lead a healthy life.
One Low Price: $14.95
Order #4810-01

Diabetes Meal Planning on $7 a Day—or Less
Patti B. Geil, MS, RD, FADA, CDE
Tami A. Ross, RD, CDE

You can save money—lots of it—without sacrificing what's most important to you: a healthy variety of great-tasting meals. Learn how to save money by planning meals more carefully, use shopping tips to save money at the grocery store, eat at your favorite restaurants economically, and much more. Each of the 100 quick and easy recipes includes cost per serving and complete nutrition information to help you create a more cost-conscious, healthy meal plan.

One Low Price: $12.95
Order #4711-01

Meditations on Diabetes
Catherine Feste

Modern medicine has come full circle to realize again what ancient healers knew: that illness affects both the body and the soul. Cathy Feste has lived with diabetes for 40 years, so she knows the physical, emotional, and spiritual challenges that come with diabetes. With every turn of the page you'll discover reassuring advice and insight in daily meditations from the author's journals with a little help from her friends, such as Ralph Waldo Emerson, Eleanor Roosevelt, Helen Keller, and many others.

One Low Price: $13.95
Order #4820-01

When Diabetes Hits Home
Wendy Satin Rapaport, LCSW, PsyD

A reassuring exploration of the full spectrum of emotional issues you and your family may struggle with throughout your lives. You'll learn how to cope with the initial period of anger and anxiety at diagnosis, develop your spiritual self and discover the meaning of living with a chronic disease, address the changes all families go through and learn how to cope with them emotionally, and much more.

One Low Price: $19.95
Order #4818-01

The Uncomplicated Guide to Diabetes Complications
Edited by Marvin E. Levin, MD
and Michael A. Pfeifer, MD

Thorough, comprehensive chapters cover everything you need to know about preventing and treating diabetes complications—in simple language that anyone can understand. All major complications and special concerns are covered, including kidney disease, heart disease, obesity, eye disease and blindness, impotence and sexual disorders, hypertension and stroke, neuropathy and vascular disease, and more.

One Low Price: $18.95
Order #4814-01

NEWLY REVISED!

Women & Diabetes, 2nd Edition
Laurinda M. Poirier, RN, MPH, CDE
Katherine M. Coburn, MPH
Special thoughts to help a woman with diabetes move through life with confidence.
One Low Price: $14.95
Order #4907-02

Caring for the Diabetic Soul
Simple solutions for coping with the psychological challenges of diabetes.
Nonmember: $9.95
Member: $8.95
Order #4815-01

Winning with Diabetes
Inspiring true stories of people who live life to the fullest, despite having diabetes.
One Low Price: $12.95
Order #4824-01

Dear Diabetes Advisor
Michael A. Pfeifer, MD, CDE
Solid, no-nonsense answers to commonsense questions about diabetes.
Nonmember: $9.95
Member: $8.95
Order #4813-01

REVISED BESTSELLER!

Type 2 Diabetes: Your Healthy Living Guide, 2nd Edition
A thorough guide to staying healthy with type 2 diabetes.
Nonmember: $16.95
Member: $14.95
Order #4804-01

Commonsense Guide to Weight Loss
Barbara Caleen Hansen, PhD
Shauna S. Roberts, PhD
Learn how to lose weight—and keep it off—using medically proven techniques from the weight-loss experts. You'll discover the seven crucial elements of weight loss for people with diabetes, including how to choose the right target weight; make permanent lifestyle changes; measure weight-loss progress by tracking health, not weight; develop a healthy meal plan; maintain an active lifestyle and more.
One Low Price: $19.95
Order #4816-01

Complete Weight Loss Workbook
Judith Wylie-Rosett, EdD, RD
Charles Swencionis, PhD
Arlene Caban, BS
Allison J. Friedler, BS
Nicole Schaffer, MA
Proven techniques for controlling weight-related health problems. The authors devised a unique workbook that offers a series of checklists, worksheets, mini-cases, calculation exercises, mental reminders, and other practical aids to knocking off those extra pounds and staying fit for good. Features real-life examples of people who illustrate and explain the patterns that lead to success or failure in watching your weight.
One Low Price: $17.95
Order #4812-01

BESTSELLER!

Diabetes & Pregnancy
Learn about an unborn baby's development, tests to expect, labor and delivery and more.
Nonmember: $9.95
Member: $8.95
Order #4903-01

Order Toll-Free: 1-800-232-6733